Childhood Uveitis

C. Stephen Foster
Luis Alonso Gonzalez-Gonzalez
Stephen D. Anesi
Suzanne Katrina V. Palafox

Childhood Uveitis

ISBN: 978-1-7332376-1-1

(Also available in eBook format.)

To The Children
And to my grandchildren:
Abigail Caroline Foster
Carson Marc Foster
Charles Matthew Foster

Preface

Uveitis is one of the leading causes of blindness worldwide. It is the third leading cause of preventable blindness in the United States. Prompt treatment of uveitis is critical to prevent visual loss and, thus, deterioration in the patient's quality of life. In addition to this, ocular inflammation does not only have a physical impact but also economical and psychological. We now know that untreated or undertreated uveitis will negatively affect the patient's life. Therefore it is of utmost importance to comprehend that the MISSION is REMISSION.

In order to understand the scope of the problem and the steps to be taken to prevent blindness in those affected by uveitis, it is important to review the classification and nomenclature of the disease. The Standardization of Uveitis Nomenclature Working Group (SUN) refined the anatomical and descriptive classification of uveitis as well as the grading system in 2005 in an effort to codify a universal language to classify ocular inflammation[1].

We convened a group of experts in Ocular Immunology and Rheumatology in an effort to provide guidelines in the diagnosis and treatment of uveitis in children. The result of this effort is captured in this monograph. The purpose of this book is to provide a concise but precise consensus on the impact of uveitis in children and on the diagnostic and therapeutic approaches.

The first chapters of this monograph describe the epidemiology, classification, nomenclature, differential diagnoses and impact on visual disability of childhood uveitis. The following chapters address diagnosing and treating Juvenile Idiopathic Arthritis associated uveitis, which represents the predominant cause of uveitis in children. Emphasis is on the rheumatologist and ophthalmologist perspectives on childhood ocular inflammation. Finally, we analyze the progress (or lack of it) achieved over the past 20 years, stressing new therapeutic insights on pediatric uveitis.

Reference:

1. Jabs DA, Nussenblatt RB, Rosenbaum JT; Standardization of Uveitis Nomenclature (SUN) Working Group. Standardization of uveitis nomenclature for reporting clinical data. Results of the First International Workshop. *Am J Ophthalmol.* 2005 140(3):509-16

Table of Contents

Chapter 1
Epidemiology: The Magnitude of the Problem

C Michael Samson MD, MBA

To understand the impact of uveitis in children, one must review the basics of epidemiology. By definition epidemiology is the study of incidence and prevalence of disease in human populations as well as their determinant factors. Defining how many children are affected by uveitis will let us understand the impact of uveitis on the society and on the individual. Moreover, comprehension of how uveitis behaves in children it is critical to establish the severity and the need of treatment. Ophthalmologists and Rheumatologists must be aware of how often the disease is chronic, how often children need to move forward to immunomodulatory therapy, how often do children develop complications from uveitis, and what is the visual outcome in children with uveitis.

There are about 30 to 40 epidemiology studies in uveitis in the literature. Unfortunately, it is difficult to come to firm conclusions given the lack of standardization of definitions and measured outcomes. In 2005 the uveitis community came to a consensus in standardizing definitions and outcome measures for the purpose of reporting clinical studies in uveitis. This was done by the Standardization Uveitis Nomenclature group[1]. However, most of the epidemiological studies occurred before 2005, thus making data interpretation difficult. Additionally when one examines the population of children affected by uveitis reported in the literature we realize that we are looking at tertiary referral centers, specializing in uveitis. This produces a referral bias that affects the interpretation of the severity of the disease. Finally, patients and populations of patients change from one epidemiological study to another based on the different regions of the world and the different time periods of the studies. Defining the magnitude of uveitis in children is a challenging quest.

There are two main epidemiologic studies reported from the United States. One was done during the 1950's and 1960's in Minnesota[2]; the other is the most recent one and is considered the largest epidemiological study in uveitis. This is the Northern California Epidemiology Uveitis Study (NCEUS)[3]. This study took advantage of the Kaiser Permanente Healthcare System, which is a health organization that provides care to one third of the population in Northern California. This epidemiology study had an opportunity of capturing all patients in a defined period of time, in this case, 12 months, thus enabling investigators to determine incidence and prevalence of uveitis.

Incidence is defined as the number of new cases of a disease in a certain population over a defined period of time (e.g. number of new cases per year in a defined population). Prevalence is the number of existing cases at any given time. The duration of a disease could be inferred by the ratio of prevalence to incidence. The NCEUS reported an incidence of 6.9/100,000 of uveitis in children. Specifically, they reported 9 new cases of uveitis in 131,802 children (ages 0-14)[3] during the year. One must carefully interpret the results of this study as prevalence and incidence are reported to be equal. Assuming that the formula for estimating the duration of a disease, according to the NCEUS, uveitis in children would have a duration of 1 year. This is clearly not what is reported in other studies. Thus, NCEUS may be valid for assessing incidence but prevalence must be interpreted with great care.

In the 1980s, an excellent study was performed in Finland. At that time all eye care was referred to one center, which made this the ideal scenario for a study in epidemiology. The researchers reported an incidence of uveitis in children of 4.3/100,000 patients and a prevalence of

27.9/100,000[4]. Incidence is approximately what the NCEUS suggests, confirming what previous studies reported. The prevalence/incidence ratio estimated a disease duration of approximately 7 years. This is more consistent with what has been reported in the literature. However, the Finland study reported 90% of uveitis to be anterior and 36% to be associated with JIA[4]. This difference in the distribution of uveitis compared to other epidemiologic studies could be explained by a regional bias due to recruiting patients from one region, Finland.

Estimating uveitis impact in children

Analyzing and considering in detail both studies, one might estimate how many children are affected by uveitis in the United States. According to the 2009 US Census data, there are about 67 million children below age 14. Considering the Finland study we could estimate that approximately 4,623 children will be diagnosed with uveitis in the USA each year. Prevalence estimation would be 30,016 children affected by uveitis in US at any one time. One way to validate this estimation is to consider that if the reported prevalence of JIA is 300,000, and 5 to 10% of these children will develop active uveitis, then about 15 to 30 thousand cases of uveitis will be seen in children. This is a good correspondence with our estimation.

One might think that 30,000 patients in a country with a population of 300 is not a big problem. However, it is indeed a very significant problem. Health care professionals must understand the laws of supply and demand and the impact of a disease on society.

Supply and demand: the impact of a disease

There are several ways to measure the impact of a disease in a society. Consider the following questions: who will take care of children affected by uveitis? Are there enough specialists who are comfortable in managing the patients? To answer these questions, a brief survey at the

New York Eye and Ear Infirmary was conducted. This showed that only 3 of 104 ophthalmologists feel comfortable in managing uveitis. The three of them were previously trained in uveitis fellowships. Moreover, only 8 of the 104 ophthalmologists reported feeling confident to surgically manage these patients. This survey also showed that less than half of ophthalmology training programs in the US have formal training in uveitis. Clearly, it is critical to educate and train more ophthalmologists to manage uveitis to supply the demand of care.

How many uveitis specialists would be necessary to provide care to all affected patients in the United States? To answer this question we will assume that all the children see a uveitis specialist, that each child is seen no more frequently than every 6 weeks, that children represent 10% of the specialist's practice and that uveitis specialists see about 160 patient visits per week. Thus, if there are approximately 30,000 affected children, the number of uveitis specialists required in the US to manage this population is about 312 uveitis specialists.

Overall, the magnitude of the number of children with uveitis is exacerbated by the lack of supply of specialists specifically trained and experienced in managing these complicated cases.

Severity of uveitis in children.

The information we have on the severity of uveitis in children is from case series from different uveitis specialty services. Smith and colleagues reported in 2009 an epidemiologic study of 527 pediatric uveitis patients from three different centers (NIH, Oregon and Chicago)[5]. Kump and collaborators published in 2004 their analysis of 269 pediatric uveitis patients over an 18 year period from a single center6. When analyzing the information reported by both studies, it is striking that up to 87% of affected children have a chronic or recurrent disease. Moreover, referral to uveitis specialists was delayed up to 6 years, and this correlated with the complication rate and visual outcome.

These studies also have shown that 32.6% of children with uveitis will require systemic immunomodulatory threapy and that many patients may suffer from vision loss in spite of aggressive treatment[5,6]. Vision loss usually occurs due to complications from uveitis. The top complications include synechiae (33.8%), *(Figure 1)* band keratopathy (20.8%), *(Figure 2)* and cataract (19.9%). The most serious are macular edema and hypotony. The complication rate increased proportionately with the duration of disease and delayed referral to specialist.

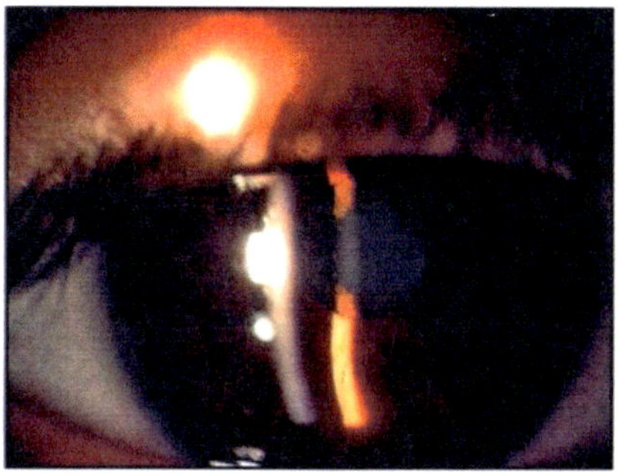

Figure 1

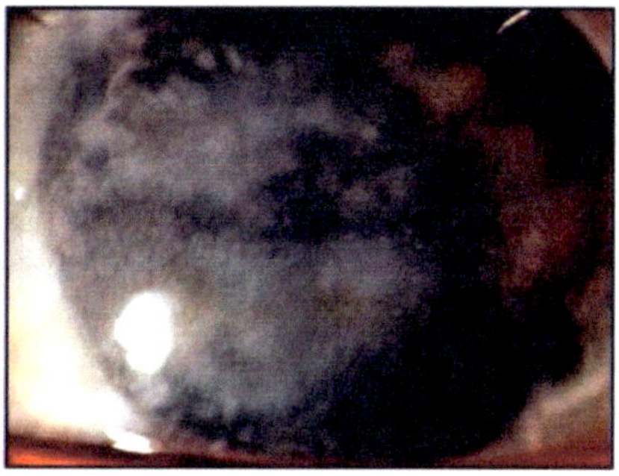

Figure 2

Unfortunately, uveitis in children still has a devastating impact in our society. The prevalence of legal blindness is around 8%-9.23%[5,6]. Although this is lower than previous reports, we need to educate and advocate to further reduce this. The socioeconomic impact of vision loss at a young age is magnified because of time; consider that the main two causes of preventable blindness in those under the age of 60 are diabetes mellitus and uveitis. Moreover, it is the lack of disease control which associates with higher rate of bilateral vision loss.

Training of qualified specialists to manage pediatric uveitis and education to ophthalmologists, rheumatologists and general population in how to early detect and refer children with uveitis is critical to prevent blindness. Early diagnosis, aggressive therapy and disease control are of utmost relevance to decrease the impact of blindness due to pediatric uveitis.

References:

1. Jabs DA, Nussenblatt RB, Rosenbaum JT; Standardization of Uveitis Nomenclature (SUN) Working Group. Standardization of uveitis nomenclature for reporting clinical data. Results of the First International Workshop. *Am J Ophthalmol.* 2005; 140(3):509-16.
2. Darrell RW, Wagener HP, Kurland LT. Epidemiology of uveitis. Incidence and prevalence in a small urban community. *Arch Ophthalmol.* 1962;68:502–14
3. Gritz DC, Wong IG. Incidence and prevalence of uveitis in Northern California; the Northern California Epidemiology of Uveitis Study. *Ophthalmol* 2004;111(3):491-500
4. Päivönsalo-Hietanen T, Tuominen J, Saari KM. Uveitis in children: population-based study in Finland. *Acta Ophthalmol Scand.* 2000;78(1):84-8
5. Smith JA, Mackensen F, Sen HN, Leigh JF, Watkins AS, Pyatetsky D, Tessler HH, Nussenblatt RB, Rosenbaum JT, Reed GF, Vitale S, Smith JR, Goldstein DA. Epidemiology and course of disease in childhood uveitis. *Ophthalmol* 2009;116(8):1544-51
6. Kump LI, Cervantes-Castañeda RA, Androudi SN, Foster CS. Analysis of pediatric uveitis cases at a tertiary referral center. *Ophthalmol.* 2005;112(7):1287-92.

Chapter 2

Standard Classification: Causes of Childhood Uveitis and Differential Diagnosis

Howard H Tessler MD

The etiology of uveitis encompasses a broad spectrum of disease. Uveitis may be a manifestation of an entity limited to the eye or of a potentially disabling or life-threatening systemic disease (cancer, auto-immune diseases). Anatomic location, type of inflammation and specific ophthalmologic findings are of utmost help when approaching uveitis. Therefore, one must systematically classify and describe the signs of the uveitis.

1. Standard of Uveitis Nomenclature and Classification[1]

1.1 Anatomical location

The same categories of uveitis that occur in adults also occur in children. **Anterior uveitis** refers to inflammation that occurs mainly in the anterior chamber and anterior vitreous. A spillover to the anterior vitreous might also be observed; this is not considered as intermediate uveitis if the cells are more abundant in the anterior segment than in the vitreous[1]. Moreover, patients with anterior uveitis may have associated cystoid macular edema and disc edema, but since these are secondary to anterior segment inflammation the inflammation is classified anatomically as an anterior.

Intermediate uveitis is a term used to describe inflammation that presents mostly in the vitreous; inflammatory cells are often seen in the anterior and peripheral vitreous[1]. Intermediate uveitis is frequently associated with peripheral vascular sheathing and cystoid macular edema. The presence of either does not change the anatomical classification, as the inflammation is located in the pars plana[1].

Posterior uveitis is inflammation that occurs in the retina or choroid[1]. Spillover of inflammatory cells into the vitreous and anterior chamber occurs in some of these patients.

Pan-uveitis refers to inflammation that appears to involve all the structures of the eye. Inflammation must be observed in the anterior segment, vitreous, retina or choroid[1]. Cystoid macular edema and neovascularization are not considered synonyms of pan-uveitis as they may also occur in anterior, intermediate, and posterior uveitides.

1.2 Clinical course of uveitis

It is important to describe the onset, duration and course of ocular inflammation when diagnosing and treating uveitis. Onset must be described as sudden or insidious; sudden onset inflammation is often self-limited and goes into remission, whereas insidious disease may last for years and either improve or worsen over time[1]. Duration of uveitis is defined as either limited, lasting 3 months or less, or persistent, lasting more than 3 months[1]. Finally, the course of uveitis must be described in terms of onset and duration. Acute disease refers to sudden and limited uveitis, while chronic uveitis encompasses insidious and persistent inflammation without episodes of inactivity. Recurrent uveitis is often referred as repeated episodes of inflammation with periods of inactivity without treatment that last more than 3 months[1]. Clinically, acute disease often presents with pain, redness and photophobia. The patient is well-aware that a problem is occurring. Chronic disease may cause vague symptoms such as floaters, light flashes (photopsias) and blurred vision the onset of which may not be readily apparent to the patient.

1.3 Granulomatous and non-granulomatous

Granulomatous is a histopathologic term that is used to characterize the clinical appearance of uveitis. Without histopathologic confirmation, this usage of the term granulomatous is not theoretically correct. However, certain types of keratic precipitates, iris nodules, vitreous cellular clumps (snowballs), retinal and choroidal lesions have been studied histopathologically and found to be granulomatous. Thus, we use the term granulomatous and non-granulomatous as a useful clinical description of the appearance of the ocular inflammation. There is no general consensus on how to classify granulomatous versus non-granulomatous and a standard reference is being develop by a panel of experts[1].

1.4 Grading inflammation

Consensus was achieved regarding a grading scheme for anterior chamber cells and flare. Inflammatory cells and flare are graded with a field size of 1mm by 1mm slit beam. See Table 1 and Table 2.

Table 1. The SUN Working Group Grading Scheme for Anterior Chamber Cells[1]

Grade	Cells in field
0+	<1
0.5+	1-5
1+	6-15
2+	16-25
3+	26-50
4+	>50

Field size: 1mm x 1mm
Adapted from reference 1

Table 2. The SUN Working Group Grading Scheme for Anterior Chamber Flare[1]	
Grade	**Cells in field**
0+	None
1+	Faint
2+	Moderate (clear details)
3+	Marked (hazy details)
4+	Severe (fibrin or plastic aqueous)
Adapted from reference 1	

We then take this terminology and apply to each clinical case and describe them with terms such as acute iridocyclitis, chronic granulomatous iridocyclitis, focal acute retinitis, granulomatous intermediate uveitis.

2. Classification of Childhood Uveitis

The incidence of pediatric uveitis is about 4.3-6/100,000 and prevalence is 20/100,000 which are 5 and 10 times lower, respectively, than in the adult population[2,3]. Due to the limitation of this article, not every type of pediatric anterior uveitis or other type of uveitis will be discussed.

Type	Entities
Anterior Uveitis	Juvenile Idiopathic Arthritis associated iritis/ iridocyclitis Acute iritis/iridocyclitis Chronic iritis of young girls Inflammatory Bowel Disease associated anterior uveitis Sarcoidosis Familial Juvenile Systemic Granulomatosis (Blau Syndrome) Herpes Simplex Virus associated uveitis Tubulointerstitial nephritis and uveitis syndrome
Intermediate Uveitis	Pars planitis Inflammatory Bowel Disease
Posterior Uveitis	Toxoplasmosis Toxocariasis

2.1 Anterior Uveitis

2.1.1 Juvenile idiopathic arthritis (JIA) associated uveitis.

This is the most common systemic disease associated with pediatric uveitis. JIA can be divided into 3 types:

1. The pauciarticular (oligoarticular) form has 4 or less joints involved in the first 6 months of onset of arthritis. This form of JIA accounts for 40-60% of all JIA cases3-5. It has been reported that 12-20% of children with this type of arthritis will develop uveitis[6].
2. The polyarticular variety of JIA presents has 5 or more joints involved and represents 40% of JIA cases. Uveitis is much less common than in the pauciarticular onset variety[3-5].
3. The systemic onset (Still's disease) type of JIA presents with fever, lymphadenopathy, rash and splenomegaly. This represents 20% of JIA cases and seldom has associated uveitis[3-5].

Pauciarticular JIA associated iritis (iridocyclitis)

These children present with 4 or fewer joints involved in the first 6 months. Later more joints can be affected. Approximately 30-50% of these patients have a monoarthritis at onset. The involved joints are asymmetric with knees and ankles most commonly involved. Many cases occur before age 6[3,7,8.] The ANA test is positive in 70-80% of cases[7,8]. Iridocyclitis has been reported in as high as 30% of these children, and occurs 4-5 times more frequently in girls than boys[8].

The onset of the iritis (iridocyclitis) is insidious and may persist for years into adulthood. These children do not have red painful eyes. (*Figure 1*) Children do not complain of blurred vision; most young children do not realize that their vision is blurred. Thus, much ocular damage can occur without parents being aware of a problem.

Uveitis in patients with JIA might begin in very young children. Up to 46% of girls who have pauciarticular, ANA positive JIA at ages 1 to 2 will develop iritis[8]. This incidence significantly drops to 10% when JIA has an onset after age 7[8].

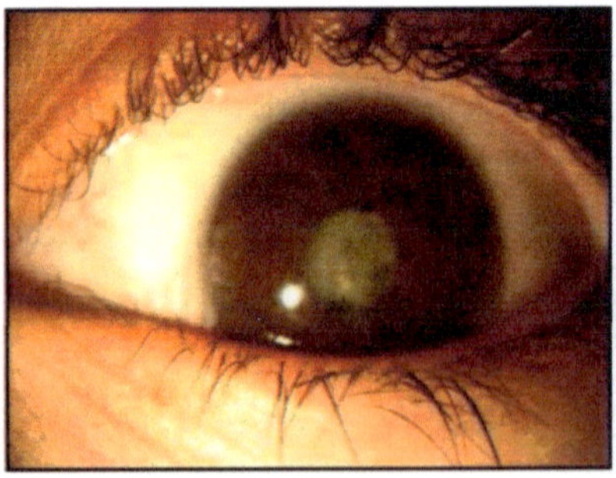

Figure 1

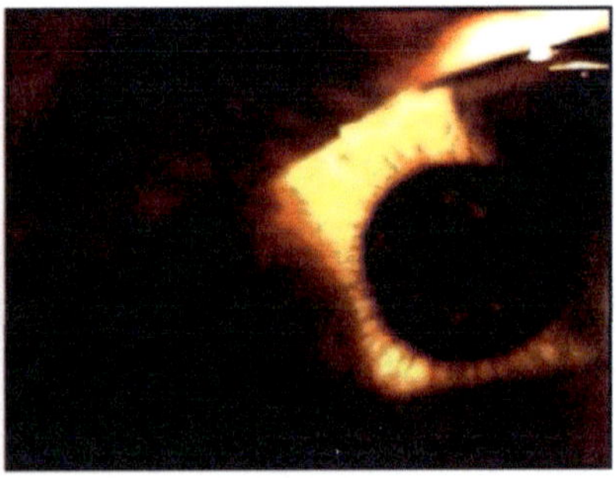

Figure 2

Given that this condition may have no symptoms, pediatricians and rheumatologists must refer these patients to ophalmologists for screening examinations. Untreated, this type of uveitis may cause permanent ocular damage such as iris synechiae, glaucoma, cataracts and phthisis bulbi. (*Figure 2*) Adherence to ophthalmologist exams is paramount in preventing damage. Data from the 1950's and 60's show that 50% of these eyes end up legally blind. To prevent blindness in these children it is mandatory to keep regular eye exam and follow directions for care.

Screening in patients with JIA

The American Academy of Pediatrics guidelines recommend that patients with high risk of developing uveitis-oligoarthritis, ANA positive and onset before age 7-be checked every 3-4 months. In most cases this involves just a rapid slit lamp examination. This frequency should be continued until at least age 12-14 when hopefully one can rely on the patient to tell us if they are aware of vitreous floaters or blurred vision. The exams could be tapered to every 6 months until age 16 and then yearly.

Medium risk children who have oligo onset arthritis and are ANA negative and have the onset of the disease at age 7 or older might be evaluated every 6 months. Finally, patients at low risk such as those with systemic onset may be assessed every 12 months.

2.1.2 Chronic Iridocyclitis of Young Girls

This disease behaves much like the chronic iridocyclitis seen in patients with JIA. However, these children have not had any arthritis. It occurs 12 times more frequently in girls than boys[8]. The same problems of management that occur with JIA associated uveitis happen with this unknown etiology type inflammation. Some of these children eventually develop arthritis. Thus, in some instances the child may have been destined to develop JIA, but uveitis developed prior to arthritis.

2.1.3 Acute Iritis and Iridocyclitis

As opposed to cases described with JIA, acute disease is very symptomatic. These children present with pain, redness and photophobia. The inflammation is usually unilateral as opposed to the bilaterality seen with JIA. Approximately 40-50% of these patients are HLA-B27 positive[9,10]; on the other hand, 16% of all pediatric anterior uveitis is related to HLA-B274. Usually this occurs in older boys at age 10 and above. Recurrences are common.

The arthritis of HLA-B27 positive children frequently involves large peripheral joints and spares the sacroiliac joints[11].

2.1.4 Inflammatory bowel disease (IBD)

Children with Crohn's disease and ulcerative colitis may develop uveitis. Uveitis is reported in 2.5% to 11% of cases of IBD[3,4]. The type of ocular inflammation seen associated with IBD includes both acute and chronic anterior uveitis as well as intermediate uveitis. Scleritis may also occur. Some patients themselves have no IBD, but give a family history of IBD and some of these patients eventually develop IBD[12].

2.1.5 Sarcoidosis

Although not common in children, about 24% to 58% of children with systemic sarcoidosis may develop uveitis[3,13]. Children younger than age 5 frequently do not have lung involvement from sarcoidosis; however, these younger patients have arthritis, rash as well as uveitis. After age 8 sarcoidosis manifests more like adult sarcoidosis with pulmonary and lymph node involvement.

Sarcoidosis in the eye is often granulomatous in appearance. The uveitis is frequently a chronic iridocyclitis but can present ubiquitously as acute iritis, intermediate uveitis, retinal periphlebitis, choroiditis, and pan-uveitis.

The diagnosis of sarcoid in someone who appears clinically only to have eye involvement can be difficult. Serum angiotensin converting enzyme (ACE) may not be a useful test given that it could be "elevated" in normal children. Serum lysozyme and chest X-rays might be of help in assessing suspected patients. Chest CT scans, although often necessary to find hilar adenopathy in adults, are usually unnecessary in children[3,13].

Finding non-caseating granulomas on biopsy is the only definitive way to establish the diagnosis of sarcoidosis. Unfortunately, there is often no easily accessible site to biopsy in children.

2.1.6 Familial Juvenile Systemic Granulomatosis (Blau syndrome)

This is a dominantly inherited condition. Patients affected by this entity have arthritis, skin lesions and chronic granulomatous uveitis and sometimes posterior uveitis. There are no pathologic findings in the lungs. This syndrome manifests exactly like sarcoidosis. Since there are cases of familial sarcoidosis one must be careful in making the diagnosis. The genetic abnormalities are located in the Nod 2-Card 15 gene.

2.1.7 Herpes simplex iritis (HSV)3

Herpes viruses are commonly overlooked cause of anterior uveitis in both children and adults. Symptoms may be vague, but HSV associated iritis usually presents acutely. Dendrite corneal lesions are clinical diagnostic of herpes but these may or may not be present. The condition is usually unilateral, with an associated elevation of the intraocular pressure, reaching 40 mm Hg in some patients. Sectoral iris atrophy with transillumination of the atrophic areas is characteristic but not always present. Spontaneous hyphema or iris hemorrhage may occur.

2.1.8 Tubular interstitial nephritis and uveitis (TINU)[15]

Patients with TINU present with bilateral anterior uveitis but onset of uveitis may be asymmetrical, with the second eye involved a week later.

It has been reported in 10% of patients presenting with bilateral anterior uveitis. Moreover, up to 32% of bilateral acute anterior uveitis in patients less than age 20 is reported to be due to TINU.

The diagnosis may be difficult is that patients are frequently unaware they have kidney disease. In tubular disease the tubules cannot reabsorb β-2 microglobulin; thus, an elevated urinary β-2 microglobulin test is highly suggestive of TINU in the setting of bilateral uveitis. Some patients with sarcoid may have renal involvement and a TINU-like picture. Although uveitis is limited and usually does not recur, uveitis may become chronic and persist for months in a small subset of these patients.

2.1.10 General work-up of anterior uveitis

A detailed, complete clinical history is invaluable. A history of red swollen joints, a family history of inflammatory bowel disease, a recent viral illness, a rash, are all positive findings which can be helpful in directing the evaluation. We usually obtain an FTA-ABS in all patients. Although syphilis is rare in children, it is a curable form of uveitis and should never be forgotten. The other lab tests should be directed as to the suspected etiology.

Chronic anterior uveitis work-up

For patients with chronic uveitis, we suggest requesting: ANA, ACE, serum lysozyme, a chest x-ray if sarcoid is suspected, a quantiferon gold (PPD) and a urinary β-2 microglobulin.

Acute anterior uveitis work-up

If acute and unilateral, order HLA-B27, but always keep HSV in mind as a possible cause. On rare occasions one might consider an anterior chamber paracentesis and PCR of the aqueous humor searching for herpes viruses DNA. Gonioscopy should be performed if one is considering the possibility of an intraocular foreign body.

If the uveitis is acute and bilateral, order: urinary β-2 microglobulin, ASO titer (ask about recent viral illnesses), IBD history in patient or family.

2.2 Intermediate Uveitis

Intermediate uveitis is a common cause of pediatric ocular inflammation and accounts for 20% of pediatric cases of uveitis. The patients may be asymptomatic, but usually complain of blurred vision and floaters. *(Figures3 and 4)*.

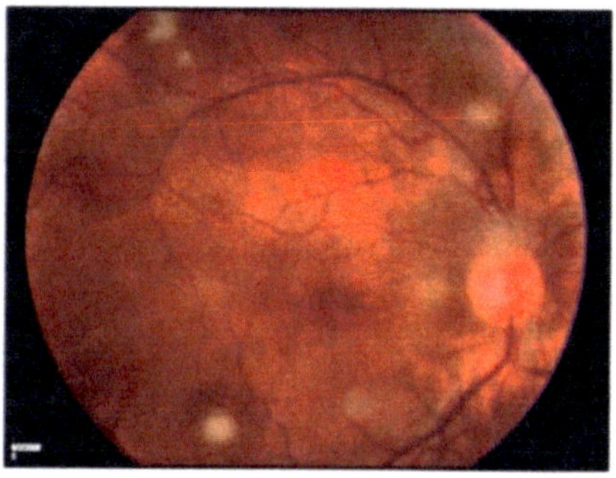

Figure 3

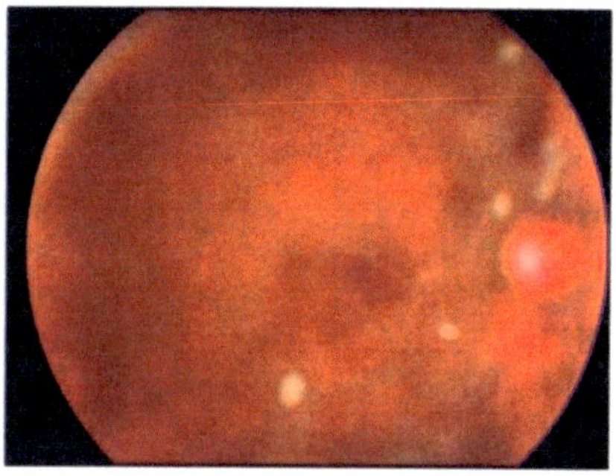

Figure 4

The eyes do not appear red or inflamed. The most common cause of intermediate uveitis is idiopathic (pars planitis); but sarcoidosis, multiple sclerosis and rarely Lyme disease may cause it too.

2.2.1 Pars Planitis (PP)[16]

This condition usually occurs in teenagers and young adults. It is chronic and frequently persists for years. It is unusual for PP to begin or persist after age 40. The incidence in Rochester MN. is 2.077/100,000 and it represented 10.9% of uveitis cases reported from St. Louis.

In young children, PP can have an active anterior uveitis component with the formation of synechia, making it appear to be a chronic iridocyclitis. Retinal vasculitis might also be associated with pars planitis *(Figures 5 and 6)*. Therapy should be individualized. Associated vasculitis often requires more aggressive therapy. The most common cause of blindness in patients with pars planitis is cystoid macular edema. To successfully treat cystoid macular edema in these patients, inflammation control must be achieved first.

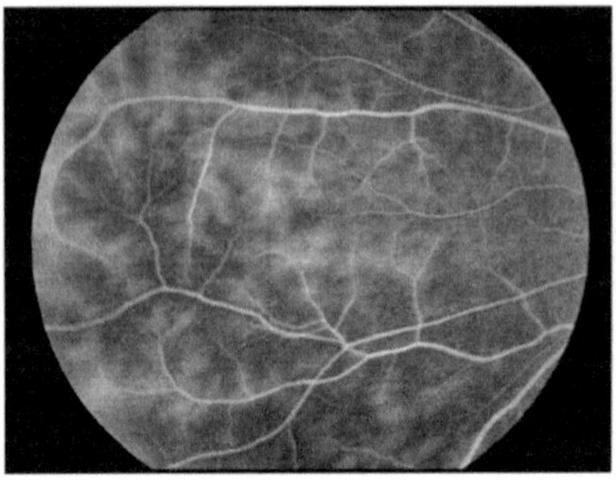

Figure 5

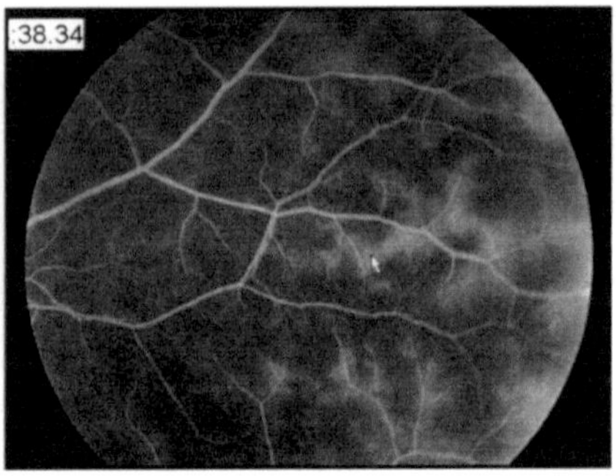

Figure 6

2.2.2 Work-up of Intermediate Uveitis

Considering etiologies other than idiopathic intermediate uveitis, we suggest requesting serum ACE, serum lysozyme, possibly a chest x-ray and a QuantiFERON®-TB Gold or PPD and Lyme titers.

2.3 Posterior Uveitis

2.3.1 Toxoplasmosis[3,17]

This is the commonest infectious cause of posterior uveitis in immunologically competent people. It is also the most common cause of posterior uveitis. It is caused by the protozoan parasite *Toxoplasma gondii.* Current seroprevalence of infection in the USA by this parasite is 22.5%. Approximately 2% of infected people have ocular disease. The incidence of toxoplasmosis is decreasing in the USA. In fact, among 12 to 49 year olds, the IgG antibody detection rate was 14.1% (1988-94) and now is 9% (1999-2004)[17].

Humans can be infected by *T. gondii* in several ways. Infection might be congenital or acquired. Congenital toxoplasmosis occurs in 1 in 10,000 births in the USA. Clinical manifestations depend on the gestational age at which infection occurred. If infection with *T.gondii* occurs during the first trimester of pregnancy, the fetus is usually aborted; in the second trimester the infant may be born with hepatosplenomegaly, lymphadenopathy, petechiae, myocarditis, encephalitis and retinochoroiditis; and, infection during the third trimester might result in a normal appearing child. However, some of these infected children will develop retinitis in later childhood or in their teens. The protozoan parasite remains viable and encysted in the retina for life.

Toxoplasmosis may also be acquired by ingesting food contaminated with oocysts. Usually this is transmitted feco-orally by eating contaminated, undercooked infected meat, particularly pork and mutton. Felines are the definitive host for *Toxoplasma gondii*, whose oocysts are shed during defecation. Children who play in soil and sandboxes contaminated with cat feces may easily acquire infection. In countries with poor water filtration, water can be a source of infection. Infection has also been reported to occur after allograft transplantation such as heart, kidney and bone marrow. Inhalation of contaminated soil (dust) is another less common source.

The hallmark of ocular toxoplasmosis is a focal retinitis, with inflammation of the adjacent choroid (*Figures 7 and 8*).

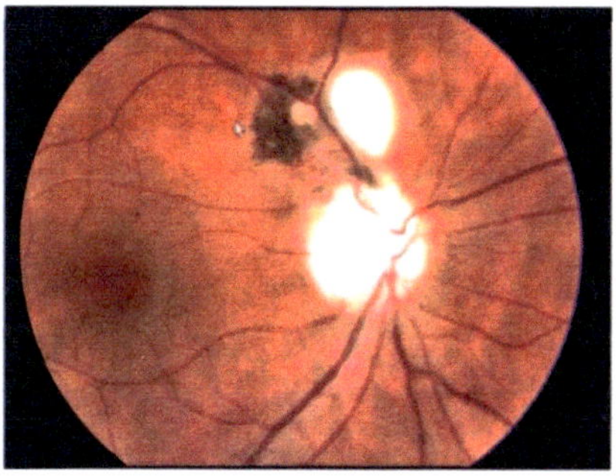

Figure 7

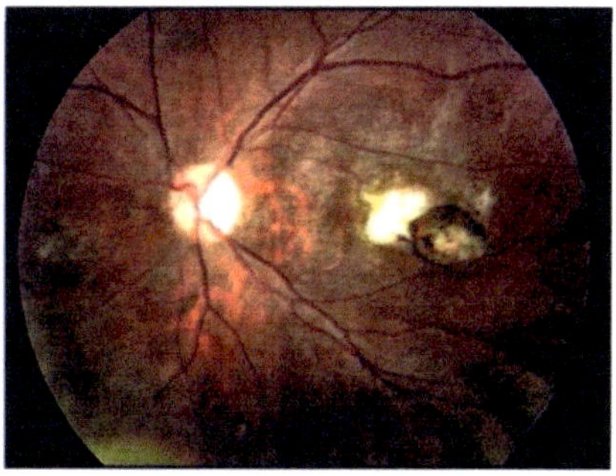

Figure 8

Frequently, the active foci of retinitis are adjacent to satellite inactive scars (*Figure 9*). Lack of previous scars should make one suspect acquired rather than congenital infection (*Figure10)*. Vitritis and anterior inflammation may occur by spillover, but the parasite is only active in the retina. Anterior uveitis might be secondary to retinal antigen exposure with subsequent autoantibodies production.

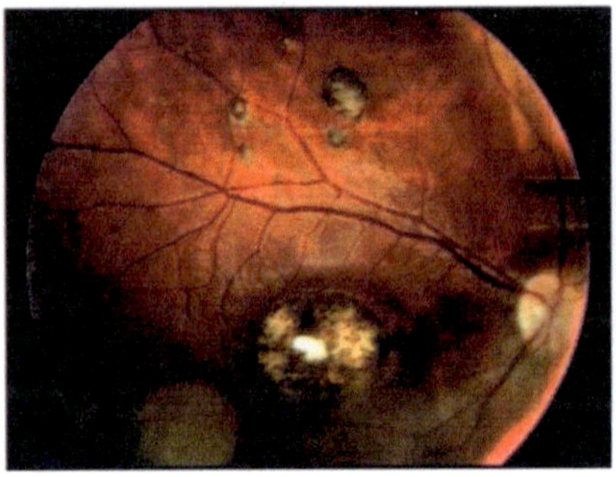

Figure 9

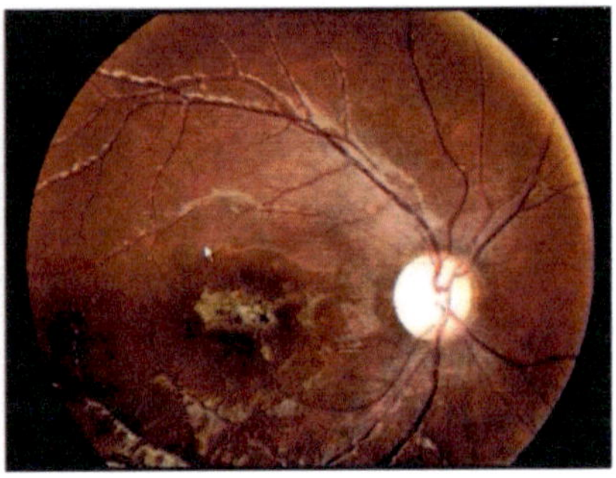

Figure 10

Toxoplasmosis work-up

Any systemic antibody titer is significant if there is a compatible fundus lesion. If the only active focus of infection is in the eye, systemic titers may be quite low. If one is uncertain as the diagnosis, an aqueous or vitreous sample can be sent for PCR analysis aimed at detecting DNA specific for *Toxoplasma gondii*. If the lesion is very characteristic, no laboratory evaluation is necessary.

2.3.2 Ocular Toxocariasis[3,18,19]

Toxocariasis is also a cause of posterior uveitis. Approximately 50% of healthy dogs may be infected with the roundworm *Toxocara canis*. Humans acquire infection by ingestion of ova contaminated soil or by contact with puppies. In fact, 28% of playground samples in Wallingford, CT were contaminated in 2005, and 25% of dogs in the UK had the roundworm ova in their hair. Moreover, ova may remain viable in soil for 25 months[18,19].

As opposed to systemic toxocariasis, patients with ocular toxocariasis usually do not have systemic signs of eosinophilic larval migrans with fever, lung involvement or high eosinophilia. The eye appears to be the only site of infection. Ocular toxocariasis is most frequently seen between ages 2 to 9, and presentation may be that of a leukocoria. Rarely there is a severe endophthalmitis, but more frequently there is a posterior pole granulomatous appearing mass or a peripheral fundus inflammatory mass in this part. Vitreous bands frequently adhere to these large solitary granulomas (*Figure 11*).

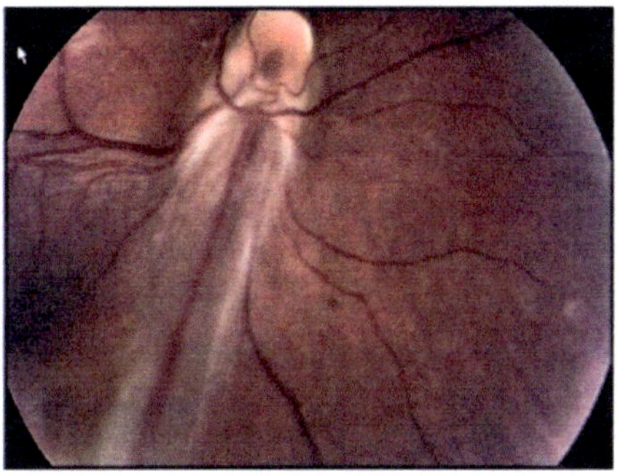

Figure 11

Toxocariasis work-up

The toxocara ELISA titer if positive is, of course, helpful. However, just as in toxoplasmosis, if the only site of infection is in the eye, systemic titers can be very low or negative. Aqueous and vitreous antibody titers should be elevated but this test may not be easy to obtain. The presence of eosinophiles on vitreous biopsy is highly suggestive of parasitic infection.

References

1. Jabs DA, Nussenblatt RB, Rosenbaum JT; Standardization of Uveitis Nomenclature (SUN) Working Group. Standardization of uveitis nomenclature for reporting clinical data. Results of the First International Workshop. *Am J Ophthalmol.* 2005 Sep;140(3):509-16.
2. Cunningham ET. Uveitis in children. *Ocul Immunol Inflamm* 2000;8:251-261.

3. Oh FS, Goldstein DA, Tessler HH. Etiologies of Pediatric Uveitis. *Contemporary Ophthalmology* 2009; 8(11):1-8
4. Patel H,Goldstein D. Pediatric uveitis. *Pediatr Clin North Am* 2003;50:125-136.
5. Kanski JJ. Juvenile arthritis and uveitis. *Surv Ophthalmol* 1990;34;253-267.
6. Keenan JD, Tessler HH, Goldstein DA. Granulomatous inflammation in juvenile idiopathic-associated uveitis. *J AAPOS* 2008;12:546-550.
7. Dana MR, Merayo-Lloves J, Schaumberg DA, Foster CS. Visual outcomes prognosticators in juvenile rheumatoid arthritis-associated uveitis. *Ophthalmol* 1997;104:236-244
8. Sauerenmann RK, Levin AV et. Al. Risk factors for the development of uveitis differ between girls and boys with juvenile idiopathic arthritis. *Arthritis Rheum* 2010; 62:1824-8.
9. Pathanapitoon K, Suksomboon S, Kunavisarut P, et al. HLA-B27-associated acute anterior uveitis in the University Referral Centre in North Thailand: clinical presentation and visual prognosis. *Br J Ophthalmol* 2006;90:1448-1450.
10. Power WJ, Rodriguez A, Pedroza-Seres M, Foster CS. Outcomes in anterior uveitis associated with the HLA-B27 haplotype. *Ophthalmology* 1998;105:1646-1651
11. Kimura SJ, Hogan MJ, O'Connor GR, Epstein WV. Uveitis and joint disease: a review of 191 cases. *Arch Ophthalmol.* 1967;77:309-16.
12. Lin P, Tessler HH, Goldstein DA. Family history of inflammatory bowel disease in patients with idiopathic ocular inflammation. *Am J Ophthalmol* 2006;141:1097-1104.
13. Shetty AK, Gedalia A. Childhood sarcoidosis: A rare but fascinating disorder. *Pediatr Rheumatol Online J.* 2008 Sep 23;6:16
14. Borzutzky A, Fried A, Chou J, Bonilla FA, Kim S, Dedeoglu F. NOD2-associated diseases: bridging innate immunity and autoinflammation. *Clin Immunol.* 2010;134(3):251-61
15. Mackensen F, Smith JR, Rosenbaum JT. Enhanced recognition, treatment and prognosis of tubulointerstitial nephritis and uveitis syndrome. *Ophthalmol* 2007;114:995-9.
16. Donaldson MJ, Pulido JS, Herman DC et al. Pars planitis: a 20-year study of incidence, clinical features and outcomes. *Am J Ophthalmol* 2007;144:812-817.
17. Jones JL, Kruszon-Moran D, Sanders-Lewis K et al. Toxoplasma gondii infection in the United States, 1999-2004, decline from the prior decade. *Am J Trop Med Hyg* 2007;77:405-10.
18. Chorazy ML, Richardson DJ, A survey of environmental contamination with ascarid ova, Wallingford, Connecticut. Vector *Borne Zoonotic Dis.* 2005;5:33-9.
19. O'Donnell CJ, Meyer KB, Jones JV et al. Survival of parasite eggs upon storage in sludge. *Appl Environ Microbiol.* 1984;48:618-25.

Chapter 3
Visual Disability in Children and Young Adults with Uveitis

David Chu MD

When a patient is visually disabled, it implies that that he or she has lost the ability to perform certain tasks because of visual impairment, generally defined by loss of visual acuity or visual field. Visual acuity is usually measured with the Snellen eye chart, or in younger pediatric patients, it can be estimated by using other devices such as the Allen picture eye chart or tumbling E chart. A person with 20/40 vision can decipher at a distance of 20 feet what a person with 20/20 vision is able to see at a distance of 40 feet. Visual field is an estimate of the spatial array of visual input and level of sensitivity that each eye, together with the brain, is able to perceive. This can be measured by several methods, including automated perimetry, where a machine creates illuminated targets a patient must acknowledge upon recognition; and tangent screen exam, where the field is tested and mapped out using targets presented by a physician or technician. A gross estimation of visual field can also be performed by confrontation finger counting when needed.

There are various definitions of visual impairment. The common definition used by doctors, nurses, schools and governmental agencies in which visually-impaired or partially-sighted is defined as vision of 20/70 or worse (best corrected) in the better eye. Legal blindness is defined as 20/200 or worse or visual field less than 20 degrees in the better eye; normal visual field is considered to be 120° horizontally. Total blindness is defined by no perception of any light.

The World Health Organization defines visual impairment in the following manner[1]:

- Low vision 1 – Best corrected vision of 20/70 or worse
- Low vision 2 – Best corrected vision of 20/200 or worse
- Blindness 3 – Best corrected vision less than 20/400 or field of 5 to 10°
- Blindness 4 – Best corrected vision less than 5/300 or field less than 5°
- Blindness 5 – No light perception

Differing types of vision loss are exemplified clinically by cataracts and glaucoma, two problems found very prominently even in the pediatric and young adult uveitic population. A patient suffering from cataracts may have diffuse blurring causing a loss of acuity. A patient with glaucoma may have excellent central acuity yet have a marked reduction in peripheral vision. In addition, color vision may be affected in eyes with glaucoma.

Visual disability implies that there is some degree of impaired functional vision, leaving a person unable to perform tasks requiring a specific level of vision. In most states, a driver must possess best corrected vision of 20/40 or better in at least one eye. In most government as well as private agencies, 20/70 or better vision is considered necessary for activities of daily living (ADL). This 20/70 mark is used by social services and schools to determine who needs special assistance.

In considering visual impairment and disability in children, one must remember that young children may not be able to voice their visual disturbance. They tend to think that everything is fine or that the way they see is normal for them. In addition, children with uveitis can and frequently do present without any noticeable symptoms or visible signs to the parents. Very young children are extremely difficult to assess as accurate vision may not be obtainable and slit-lamp examination, the method generally employed by ophthalmologists to detect intraocular inflammation, may not readily be performed. Yet making the effort to properly evaluate this population is crucial as visual disability has a greater impact over the lifetime of children and young adults because of their potential to be productive members of society.

Visual impairment is not always permanent. In many cases it is clearly reversible, as seen with pharmacologic changes (i.e. eye drops), inflammation, and cystoid macular edema (CME). CME, however, if left chronic and inadequately treated, can lead to retinal damage and permanent visual loss. Patients with cataract, corneal scarring, or retinal detachment will require surgical correction to improve their vision. When vision is lost from glaucoma, whether it is uveitic glaucoma or response to steroid, it is not recoverable. Hypotony, retinal atrophy, and amblyopia can also cause permanent visual impairment. Hypotony can especially prove difficult to treat; however, correction of intraocular pressure to normal levels in these patients at times improves vision.

Several reports evaluating large series of pediatric uveitis patients have been published since 2000. Among them, five reported data on vision levels of the subjects[2-6]. The majority of subjects presented with or developed one or more ocular complications secondary to uveitis or treatment of the uveitis, ranging from 76 to 95%[2-6]. Nineteen to 28% of subjects in these papers required one or more surgeries[2-6]. Worse visual outcomes were frequently associated with juvenile idiopathic arthritis (JIA) and pars planitis, both generally chronic in nature. The rate of visual impairment (20/50 to 20/70) at the time of presentation was approximately 30% in these five papers and the rate of legal blindness (<20/200) at the time of presentation ranged from 9-17%[2-6]. Three of five papers had data pertaining to the treatment and outcomes. Analysis of visual outcomes following treatment among institutions involved in these reports indicated that the rate of legal blindness ranged from 7-15%, implying that once the vision is altered to this level, even after diagnosis and treatment, the outcome generally is not favorable[2-6].

Foster's group reviewed 269 pediatric uveitis cases at a major tertiary care center in 2005[4] and concluded that the rate of complication was highest among JIA patients and increased with the duration of uveitis. Furthermore, they reported that as the duration of time between diagnosis of uveitis and evaluation by a uveitis specialist increased, visual outcome worsened.

In a review of 527 pediatric uveitis patients at three tertiary care centers performed by Smith et al. in 2009, visual outcome data showed CME and hypotony had the most negative impact on vision.[6] In addition, posterior uveitis and panuveitis were associated with more severe loss. They also discovered that the prevalence of pediatric patients with uveitis with compromised vision (<20/200) varies only minimally over 10 years, indicating the need for aggressive monitoring and proper treatment of children with uveitis, and the necessity to assess the impact of the disease on age-appropriate activities of daily living.

In summary, visual impairment is a common consequence in children and young adults with uveitis. Higher rates of ocular complications and worse visual impairment are generally associated with chronic disease, as well as delayed referral to uveitis specialist. Visual prognosis is favorable with appropriately aggressive and timely treatment; if significant vision loss exists at the time of presentation, it may not improve even with treatment. There is no accurate measure of true visual impairment, and when disability is implied, it means much more than just numbers. Treating the disease more effectively and efficiently, as well as education of ophthalmologists and parents, may reduce the overall rate of visual disability in these children.

References:

1. The prevention of blindness. Report of a WHO Study Group. Geneva, World Health Organization, 1973 (WHO Technical Report Series, No. 518).
2. deBoer J, Wulffraat N, Rothova A. Visual loss in uveitis of childhood; *Br J Ophthalmol* 2003;87:879-84
3. Edelsten C, Reddy MA, Stanford MR, et al. Visual loss associated with pediatric uveitis in English primary and referral centers; *Am J Ophthalmol* 2003; 123:676-80
4. Kump LI, Cervantes-Castaneda RA, Androudi AN, Foster CS. Analysis of pediatric uveitis cases at a tertiary referral center. *Ophthalmol* 2005;112:1287-92
5. Rosenberg KD, Feuer WJ, Davis JL. Ocular complication of pediatric uveitis; *Ophthalmol* 2004;111:2299-306
6. Smith JA, Friederike M, Sen HN, et al. Epidemiology and course of disease in childhood uveitis; *Ophthalmol* 2009;116:1544-51

Chapter 4
A Family Affair: Impact of parental and caregiver concerns on families coping with chronic illness

Janis Arnold

4.1 Impact of chronic illness

The impact of chronic illness is far reaching, and has a cascading effect for many family members who provided caretaking roles who have emotional investment in the child's well-being. A chronic "childhood" medical condition is a "family" medical condition. Negotiating the medical demands impacts:

- Patient
- Parents
- Marriage/partnership
- Siblings
- Extended family

Everyone affected may have varied coping mechanisms to manage living with a chronic illness. Considerations and variables that impact coping are multi-faceted.

- Differing coping styles
- Different developmental stages of family members
- Previous context/history with illness & grief
- Ambivalence between craving choices and craving guidance
- Loss

4.2 Loss

Any time there is change, there is loss; this may be loss of the previous family routine, the previous family roles, the predictability of one's body or eyesight. The natural emotional response to any loss, can be one of grief. Diagnosis and medical demands that lead to changes often lead to grieving the loss of the anticipated childhood, both for the patient and the parents. Coping with diagnosis of chronic illness can often mirror grief cycle[1], though we know these reactions are often not linear.

- Denial
- Anger
- Bargaining
- Depression
- Acceptance

4.3 Conceptual model

The biopsychosocial model is a general model or approach to chronic health conditions that posits that biological, psychological and social factors, all play a significant role in human functioning in the context of illness.

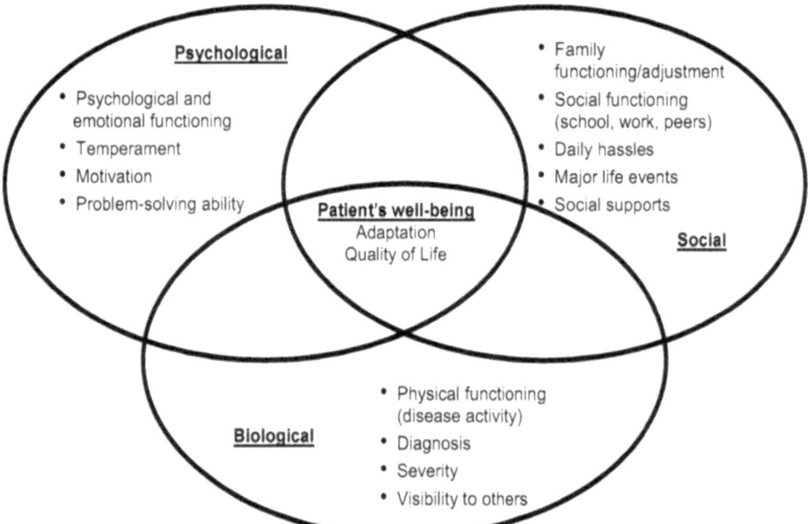

Health is best understood in terms of a combination of biological, psychological, and social factors rather than purely in biological terms.

This allows for more comprehensive appreciation of the various spheres within which a patient and family function and promotes a multidisciplinary approach to health-relate d quality of live. This conceptual model was first promoted by George Engel in 1977.

4.4 Protecting childhood

When looking at a childhood that is peppered with ongoing medical demands, one of the most essential priorities is preserving childhood. This includes helping patients forge a self-identity that includes differentiation apart from uveitis; children have uveitis, uveitis doesn't have them. It can help to do exercises that remind children of all of the other group affiliations they have, that contribute to their identity. These can include being a son/daughter, sibling, friend, student, musician, athlete, artist, and then a patient. It can be on the list, but is just one of many characteristics. In an effort to preserve childhood, it is critical to try to counter the recurrent and often primary socialization that is occurring in the adult world of medicine. Providing constant opportunities for peer play is crucial, and may take some deliberate planning.

4.5 Parent/caregiver concerns

Parents are charged with the extraordinary task of negotiating multiple concerns, variables and feelings brought about by managing chronic illness. Their goal is quality of life, but for *all* family members, which can require constant reconciliation of and shift on roles and priorities within a family system.

Caregiver concerns often include, but are not limited to:

- The typography of chronic illness: Cyclical vs. progressive
- Complications that can remit and relapse
- Unpredictablity
- Disempowerment
- Anxiety
- Confusion

- Helplessness
- Medication choices that can be dizzying at best, scary at worst
- Risks
- Cost/benefits of treatment options
- Side effects
- Lack of reliable information or data, which can lead to anxiety

We know that parents and adults often experience what child is not cognitively capable of experiencing, such as a sense of hopelessness, grief or fear. Over time, it is easy to unknowingly relocate these feelings onto other child/family members. This helps bring a caregiver validation for their feelings and invites emotional companionship on journey of chronic illness

4.6 Impact on patient

Patients have their own distinct concerns and implications of treatment. Children read adults' facial cues and tones of voice and at particular developmental stages, children will often try protect their parents from information or feelings that children may feel would be upsetting to parents. We want to allow a child to feel safe coming to caregivers and medical team member's with their own fears.

When questions arise, it is important to always answer questions honestly, even if not fully, in an effort to dispel myths. Without accurate information, children will make up their "own" story from pieces of information they collect, and this may be worse or scarier than the real story.

We want to allow child to have own feelings and prevent the tendency for over-identification with a caregivers' distinct feeling or a child's attempts to please caregivers or medical clinicians, by having what a child may think is the "right" answer or symptom report.

Adherence to the medical regimen is clearly a large part of reducing complications of uveitis. For patients, lack of information can decrease compliance, if the cost/benefit analysis for follow-through with treatment is being based on incorrect considerations or incomplete information. Loss of control over one's body or one's own right to self-determination, when a teenager is dependent on parents and physicians, can increase what often appears to defiance, when it is ambivalence.

4.7 Choices

- Offer choices whenever possible
- Regardless of seemingly insignificant decision
- Choices can be around medical or non-medical options
- Increase feelings of empowerment
- Avoid presenting choices that are too burdensome
- Don't offer a choice, when a decision not truly up to the child. When we say "should we take our medicine now?" or "want to go take to your medicine?", it seems there a couple of possible answers. It is better to ask "do you want to take you medicine now, or at the next commercial?" This is a choice that is indeed up to the child.

4.8 Preparation, anticipation, communication

These three simple things can help enhance families' ability to manage demands and increase partnerships with the medical team

- Listening, just listening, to a patient and family– this can help them identify strengths, and vulnerabilities that will impact the way they are able to navigate or cope with the medical demands and treatment
- Providing anticipatory guidance – this then allows for problem-solving barriers that may exist for next stages of treatment
- Reframing – this can help normalize their experiences

- Developing action plans
- Developing short, long term goals, do combat hopelessness and helplessness.

4.9 Considerations

With uveitis, as with any chronic illness, there are multiple considerations families reconcile on a day-to-day basis.

- "Going public"
- Making decisions - who is involved?
- Trust with providers
- Identifying support networks
- Dispelling myths
- Finding and forming mutual aid connections
- Making time for self-care

4.10 Impact on siblings

The adjustment of siblings to a "chronic illness"-a friendly home and lifestyle can often be under recognized, amidst the dizzying logistical, emotional and educational demands of the child with the medical condition.

Meeting all the needs of the child with uveitis can seem to use all the energy and focus. However, being the sibling of a child with a chronic illness can have its own effects, and with attention, can ultimately be a growth-enhancing experience. Reactions and experiences can be as unique as one's child, but there are some recurrent themes and common experiences of siblings.

- Jealousy - siblings may also want to be "sick" for increased attention
- Different access than the parents to medical explanations can lead to fear
- Guilt – why am I healthy if my brother is sick

- Resentment over unequal division of family resources/time
- Fear over their own invincibility and potential for getting a chronic illness.

Most younger children engage in magical thinking, and siblings, who often don't come to the doctor visits or have frequent access to the same explanation that parents or the child with the medical condition does, often have myths about cause and effect. Children often adjust best when they feel a sense of mastery over the information; including siblings in the daily management of the demands is a great way to involve them in the experience. It can also help prevent the sense that there is a conspiracy to keep this medical "secret" between just the parent(s) and their brother or sister.

4.11 Children's roles

Children often attempt to keep balance amidst perceived chaos; this is not always seen, but can be common ways that children inadvertently help a family keep functioning amidst a change in routine.

- Hero - successful, pressure to be responsible and uphold family's self-esteem
- Mascot - Affectionate, clown, pressure to get along, be able to laugh
- Lost child – self-contained, adaptable, detached, safety in being invisible

It is important to remember that with all these roles, children can still internalize fear or loneliness. Prompting them to share their thoughts periodically may help get through their outer "characters".

4.12 Use of language

With good intentions, caregivers and medical staff often use words and language that have multiple meanings to children. These ambiguous medical expressions can easily scare children.

- "dye" vs. "die"
- "dressing change" makes children afraid they must be naked
- "shot"
- words that are usually positive descriptors – "special", "funny" when describing how a treatment or test will feel, then making children question the meaning of the word.

4.13 Impact in school realm

School is a child's career. A chronic medical condition affecting vision requires and is entitled to protective environmental and academic accommodations within the school setting in an individualized health plan or 504 Plan under the American with Disabilities Act. If team meetings are scheduled or occurring to address these accommodations, it is important that the students know this, so they are aware advocacy is happening and can feel better supported.

Helping children anticipate and rehearse answers to peer questions is also helpful and can reduce anticipatory anxiety about how much information to provide and to whom to provide it. Questions may range from noticeable side effects of medications to absences for infusions. Having two or three prepared phrases can help patients feel less stigmatized.

Naturally, missing school for office visits, procedures or infusions (any of which could be scheduled or unscheduled) can lead to peer isolation; creating specific opportunities for peer play and socialization is important.

4.14 Developmental framework

There is a developmental framework to most things – families, individuals, marriages and partnerships, as well as the journey of living with a chronic medical condition.

Caregivers need to have an awareness of "normal" child development so that realistic expectations are conveyed to child. Then, it is important to have awareness of barriers to enabling this developmental process. The ongoing demands and dependency created by a childhood medical condition can pose potential barriers to obtaining the skill mastery in adolescence, separation/individuation, identity formation, and launching.

4.15 Developmental Considerations

The following table simply reminds us of the various individual stages of socio-emotional development and the tasks we are charged with in each stage. Chronic medical demands that occur or persist through certain stages can impact the mastery of these identified tasks. Knowing this context can help caregivers better respond to missed opportunities or create strategies to compensate for stages in which patients may be struggling.

Developmental Stage	Task	Impact
Infancy	Attachment, trust	Bonding
Toddler	Autonomy	Control
Pre-school	Initiative	Separation, regression
School age	Industry, socialization	Mastery, peer relationships
Adolescence, Young adulthood	Identity, Independence, Sexuality	Body Image, Intimacy, Achievement

4.16 Family stages of development

Similarly, family units pass through normal, expected life stages that form the family's capacity to adapt, as a social system that evolves over time, among new sets of circumstances. This can lead to shifts in family composition and the adaptability to change can promote familial resiliency.

These stages include:
1. Formation of strong partner relationship
2. Nurturance of family members
3. Individuation of family members
4. Developing partnerships outside of family
5. Regrouping (launching)
    - Main task is allowing for safe & healthy departure[2]

4.17 Building resiliency

It is indeed an ongoing process, but most families are doing this, without calling it such. The following factors can help facilitate trust in the medical system, optimism, resiliency and ultimately, health-related quality of life.

- Exploring adjustment of other family members
- Identifying the practical resources available – financial, logistical, concrete
- Effective advocacy for relevant school accommodations
- Using materials for medical play around pending medical interventions to develop childrens' sense of mastery
- Identifying social supports: groups, individual counseling, one-to-one mentoring, (as mentor or mentee), religious or faith-based networks
- Normalize feelings
- Maintain consistent routine

- Continue discipline as caregiver would with other siblings or with child without medical condition
- Probe with open-ended questions to allow own formation of thoughts/reactions

4.18 Techniques for caregivers

Strategies to help caregivers help children

- Verbalize/sort through feelings and emotional reactions generated by decisions facing family with another adult, so not inadvertently projected onto child as their fear
- Help child make own list of changes/losses, limitations – to openly distinguish child concerns as his/her own
- Teach positive self-talk statement to child ("I have uveitis, it doesn't have me"; "Uveitis is a part of me, not all of me")
- Explore misconceptions that interfere with optimal adherence by patient
- Maintain running list of activities that child can still enjoy alone or with family/peers
- Identify own cognitive distortions/negative automatic thoughts that contribute to fear, to help avoid "catastrophizing"
- Describe various coping styles of various caregivers, so that needs can be met by one another, not inadvertently taken on by child/siblings
- Increase communication, awareness and ownership of each family member's feelings through age-appropriate channels
    - Art
    - Worry jars
    - Story writing
    - Lists of "tips" for other, newly diagnosed children, which can help increase feeling of control

"Promise me you'll always remember: You're braver than you believe, and stronger than you seem, and smarter than you think."

~Christopher Robin (to Winnie the pooh)

References

1. Kübler-Ross E. *On Death and Dying,* 1969. Macmillan, NY.
2. Rhodes SL. A developmental approach to the life cycle of the family. *Social Casework* 1977;58,:301-311
3. Erickson E. (1980). *Identity and the Life Cycle.* WW Norton and Co., New York, NY.
4. Zittel KM, Lawrence S, Wodarski JS. Biopsychosocial Model of Health and Healing: Implications for Health Social Work Practice. *J Human Behavior Social Environment* 2002;5(1):19–33.

Chapter 5
Childhood Uveitis: Special Challenges

David Hinkle MD

When addressing uveitis in children one must consider the special challenges that this involves. As opposed to adults, obtaining a logical description of symptoms, realizing the ophthalmological exam and, even obtaining diagnostic tests in children pose special challenges.

5.1 Symptoms in children

Symptoms of uveitis depend on a number of factors, including age, duration, chronicity and location. It is important to consider that half of children with uveitis are asymptomatic *(Figure 1)*. When present, signs and symptoms of uveitis in children may include redness, pain, light sensitivity, blurry vision, floaters, ptosis, strabismus (although diplopia is unusual), and opacification of the cornea and ocular media *(Figure 2)*. Interestingly, band keratopathy occurs frequently in chronic forms of childhood uveitis and is present in 77% of patients with juvenile idiopathic arthritis associated uveitis.

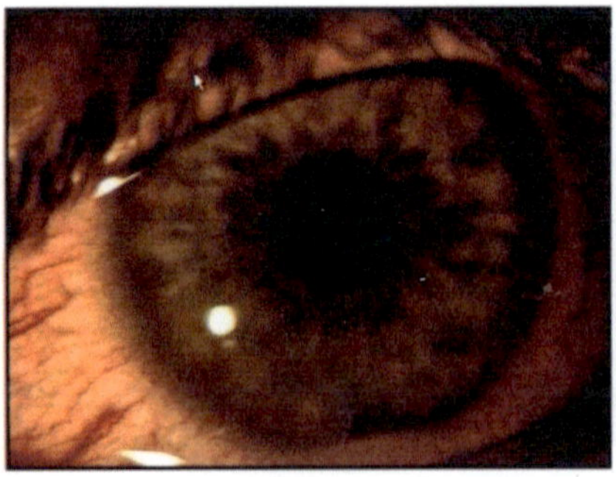

Figure 1

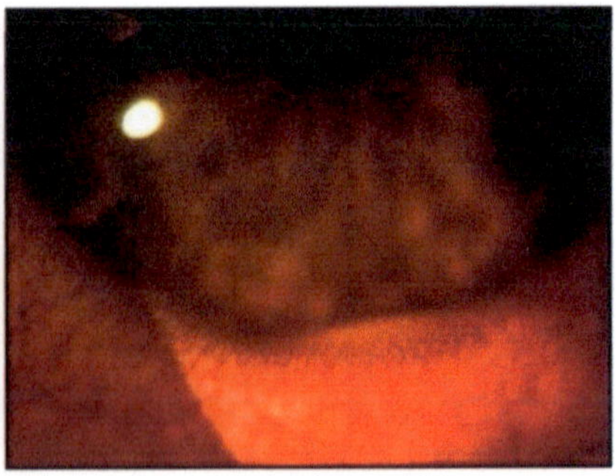

Figure 2

5.2 Vision Testing

Vision testing is an approximation in many children but is most difficult in the pre-verbal age group. Questions to answer include:

1. Does the child fix and follow? Moving a tilting a mirror in front of the child should illicit fixation movements.
2. Does the child smile toward parents and reach for objects?
3. Is fixation central, steady, and maintained?

For older, preschool age children, acuity can be tested with charts other than the standard Snellen chart. Figures, numbers, Landolt C, and tumbling E charts are particularly useful and hand held near vision cards may improve attention span.

5.3 The ophthalmologic exam

5.3.1 'Pearls' for clinical exam

Examining a child could be challenging and frustrating if proper approach is not followed. When examining a child, keep the following pearls in mind.

1. Be yourself, children can spot a phony.
2. Be honest; don't say something will not hurt when you know it will.
3. Have fun, smile, and make the encounter light and playful.
4. Remember the one toy – one look rule; have an array of age appropriate toys.
5. Greet the child and speak directly to her.
6. Examine a parent, older sibling, or stuffed animal first.
7. Go where the action is – you may only get a few moments of co operation, check what you most need to see first.
8. Abandon the white coat.
9. Wear fun ties, scarves, or other clothing children will enjoy.

10. Delegate eye drops and other unpleasant tasks to assistants.
11. Employ positive phraseology, avoid negative suggestions.
12. Abandon or repeat the examination if building rapport is more im portant.
13. Be persistent when dealing with live or vision threatening prob lems.
14. Use sedation and anesthesia if necessary.
15. Consider a pediatric area or at least some toys in the waiting room.
16. Keep finger puppets on hand.
17. Collaborate with a pediatric ophthalmologist.
18. Parents are right until proven otherwise.
19. When all else fails, consider rewards for cooperation.

5.3.2 Intraocular pressure measurement

Intraocular pressure testing is fraught with difficulties in the pediatric age group. Goldmann applanation is inaccurate in children under the age of 9 years owing to lower ocular rigidity. The Pascal Dynamic Contour Tonometer™ may be more accurate but there are few studies in children to date. Pneumotonometry is generally well tolerated and works well in cases of nystagmus. It may be used on the cornea or sclera and over contact lenses. Older models of the Tonopen™ sampled at low rates leading to inaccuracies. Newer models of both the Pneumotonometer™ and Tonopen are probably more accurate in children. The Ocular Response Analyzer™ may be a viable alternative for non-contact (air puff) tonometry although this has not been validated in children. Finally, one should not forget the value of palpation. If the globe feels like your cheek the pressure is low, like your nose the pressure is normal, like your chin the pressure is elevated.

5.3.3 The slit lamp exam

Slit lamp examination by an experienced specialist is frequently necessary to establish the diagnosis of uveitis. Grading anterior chamber reaction prior to dilation of the pupils eliminates the component of pigment release which may occur following mydriasis. Use of one of the standard grading scales is useful when communicating with other providers or for study purposes. Anterior chamber flare without cells usually does not require treatment although studies by Holland and associates are causing a re-evaluation of this axiom[1]. Laser flare photometry values correlate with a number of ocular inflammatory markers and sequelae. Elevated flare, independent of anterior chamber cells, is associated with an increased risk of vision loss and glaucoma[1]. Vitreous haze quantified according to the grading scale introduced by Nussenblatt is a more sensitive indicator of active inflammation than vitreous cells[2].

5.3.4 The physical examination

Remember to examine the joints, particularly the knees of children with uveitis. Ophthalmologists should not miss the opportunity to diagnose arthritis and make early referral to a pediatric rheumatologist.

5.4 Final remarks

The chronic nature of many forms of childhood uveitis remains a great challenge[3]. The International Uveitis Study Group defines uveitis as chronic when active for more than 3 months[3]. This is more common in females with JIA and frequently leads to band keratopathy, formation of posterior synechiae, cataracts, glaucoma and hypotony[4,5,6]. Four large retrospective studies in the past 7 years illustrate the stubborn nature of childhood uveitis[4]. The mean age at presentation to a uveitis specialist was 8-9 years with mean duration of approximately 2 years[4]. A slight female majority was observed. Surprisingly fewer than half of affected individuals had isolated anterior uveitis[4]. The vast majority of cases were bilateral with a follow-up ranging from 2-6 years[4]. A multidisciplinary approach to treatment yields the best outcomes.

References:

1. Holland GN. A reconsideration of anterior chamber flare and its clinical relevance for children with chronic anterior uveitis (an American Ophthalmological Society thesis). *Trans Am Ophthalmol Soc.* 2007;105:344-64.
2. Nussenblatt RB, Palestine AG, Chan CC, Roberge F. Standardization of vitreal inflammatory activity in intermediate and posterior uveitis. *Ophthalmol* 1985;92:467-471.
3. Smith JA, Mackensen F, Sen HN, Leigh JF, Watkins AS, Pyatetsky D, Tessler HH, Nussenblatt RB, Rosenbaum JT, Reed GF, Vitale S, Smith JR, Goldstein DA. Epidemiology and course of disease in childhood uveitis. *Ophthalmol* 2009;116:1544-51.
4. Kump LI, Cervantes-Castañeda RA, Androudi SN, Foster CS. Analysis of pediatric uveitis cases at a tertiary referral center. *Ophthalmol.* 2005;112:1287-92.
5. Rosenberg KD, Feuer WJ, Davis JL. Ocular complications of pediatric uveitis *Ophthalmol.* 2004;111:2299-306.
6. de Boer J, Wulffraat N, Rothova A.Visual loss in uveitis of childhood. *Br J Ophthalmol.* 2003;87:879-84.

Chapter 6

Pediatric Uveitis: Eye/Joint Disparate Inflammation

H. Nida Sen, MD, MHc

Pediatric uveitis constitutes about 10% of all uveitis cases. Among these, 28-58% of cases have no associated systemic disease and 20-33% have associated juvenile idiopathic arthritis (JIA). Thus, JIA is the most common associated systemic disease in childhood uveitis. Approximately 30-35% of all JIA cases develop uveitis (ranges between 15 to 45% in different series). JIA prevalence in the U.S. is estimated at 113.4 per 100,000 (95% CI 54.6, 155.1) and each year[1], between 7,157 and 13,590 are children expected to develop JIA nationwide[2]. There are between 39,470 and 112,130 children with JIA in the U.S. Since 15-30% of all JIA cases develop uveitis, there are ~12,000 to 30,000 kids with JIA- associated uveitis in the U.S. with at least two thousand new JIA-associated uveitis cases each year.

Different classifications have been used by different groups to define the joint involvement in JIA. The American College of Rheumatology (ACR) simply describes 3 categories of JIA (previously juvenile rheumatoid arthritis, JRA): 1) Pauciarticular, 2) polyarticular and 3) systemic onset JIA. EULAR (The European League Against Rheumatism) and ILAR (International League of Associations for Rheumatology) use a slightly different nomenclature. Pauciarticular JIA constitutes 80-90% of patients with JIA-associated uveitis, polyarticular JIA constitutes 7-14%, and systemic onset JIA less than 1-5%. This already shows the discordance between the joint involvement and the eye inflammation; pauciarticular exceedingly more commonly associated with uveitis while polyarticular JIA with more joint involvement is much less often associated with ocular inflammation. While the type of JIA confers a risk for ocular involvement, the course, severity and timing of joint involvement in a particular patient often has no relation to the ocular inflammation.

The initial presentation of disease varies greatly as well. The average age of onset of uveitis in children with JIA is 6 yrs and uveitis typically develops within 5 to 7 yrs of onset of arthritis. In 60% arthritis antedates uveitis (1-6 yrs)[3], in 25-30% of cases both are diagnosed simultaneously and in 10-13% uveitis antedates joint manifestations (~1 year). Multiple studies have shown differences in the course of joint disease and eye disease since the 1980s. Rosenberg and colleagues showed in a series of 35 patients with JIA and uveitis with long-term follow-up that in 70% of patients the patterns of joint and eye activity differed3. For example, there were patients with relapsing and remitting joint disease who had a single episode of uveitis, whereas some patients with a single episode of arthritis suffered from unremitting eye disease. They also reviewed the literature with similar series and concluded that approximately 78% of cases had either eye or joint activity when the other was deemed inactive[3].

The differential response to certain immunomodulatory treatments also supports this discordant activity in joints and eyes. Etanercept, an IgG antibody engineered against TNF, has been found to be quite effective for arthritis but not as effective in controlling ocular inflammation. In two double-masked, randomized clinical trials of etanercept for treating JIA-associated uveitis, one by Foster and colleagues[4] and the other conducted at the National Eye Institute (NEI)[5], etanercept was no more effective than placebo. In another pilot open-label study for the treatment of JIA-associated uveitis at the NEI[6], daclizumab, a monoclonal antibody directed against the IL-2 receptor on T cells, was used to control active ocular inflammation with relative success in most cases. However despite the quiescence of the eye disease one patient showed a dramatic flare-up of systemic and joint disease while on therapy. These are just a few examples of the overwhelming evidence of the discrepancy between the eye and joint inflammation in children with JIA-associated uveitis.

Discordant inflammation in the joints and eyes in JIA and JIA-associated uveitis suggests that, although a common etiologic factor may be responsible for both manifestations, the pathogenesis leading to the initiation and recurrence of activity is different. Understanding of the pathogenesis of the ocular inflammatory response during active uveitis and how it differs from that of associated arthritis may facilitate the identification and evaluation of other immunosuppressive or immunomodulatory strategies for treatment of JIA-associated uveitis.

References:

1. Towner SR, Michet CJ, O'Fallon WM, Nelson AM. The epidemiology of juvenile arthritis in Rochester, Minnesota, 1960-1979. *Arthritis Rheum.* 1983;26:1208-13.
2. Bowyer SL, et al. Health status of patients with juvenile rheumatoid arthritis at 1 and 5 years after diagnosis. *J Rheumatol.* 2003 Feb;30(2):394-400.
3. Rosenberg AM, et al. The relationship between ocular and articular disease activity in children with juvenile rheumatoid arthritis and associated uveitis. *Arthritis Rheum.* 1986 29(6): 797-800.
4. Foster CS, et al. Efficacy of etanercept in preventing relapse of uveitis controlled by methotrexate. *Arch Ophthalmol.* 2003 Apr; 121(4): 437-40.
5. Smith JA et al. A randomized, placebo-controlled, double-masked clinical trial of etanercept for the treatment of uveitis associated with juvenile idiopathic arthritis. *Arthritis.* 2005;53, (1):18-23
6. Sen HN, et al. High-dose daclizumab for the treatment of juvenile idiopathic arthritis-associated active anterior uveitis. *Am J Ophthalmol.* 2009;148(5):696-703
7. Gallagher M, Quinones K, Cervantes-Castañeda RA, Yilmaz T, Foster CS. Biological response modifier therapy for refractory childhood uveitis. *Br J Ophthalmol.* 2007 Oct;91(10):1341-4.

Chapter 7
A Rheumatologist's Perspective on Childhood Uveitis

Patrick Whelan MD PhD

The year 2010 marks the hundredth anniversary of the first report, by a German ophthalmologist named Johannes Ohm, of uveitis (in that case, iridocyclitis and band keratopathy) in a girl with chronic arthritis.[1] He reported the case without a conviction that the two conditions were directly related, but a string of case reports followed and the matter became settled with the first case series published in the 1950s.[2] Dr Jane Schaller, the distinguished pediatric rheumatologist who chaired the Pediatrics Department at Tufts/New England Medical Center, appreciated in the 1960s that children with JIA and a positive blood test for anti-nuclear antibodies (ANA) had a higher likelihood of developing uveitis.[3]

Dr Stephen Foster and colleagues have since published a number of papers suggesting that juvenile idiopathic arthritis, more than other causes of uveitis, predisposes to loss of vision if inadequately treated. JIA is also among the most common causes of uveitis. About one-third of the eyes in children with JIA-associated uveitis develop visual impairment, and one in ten become legally blind.[4] Predicting visual prognosis in these patients appears most closely correlated with (1) either onset of uveitis prior to arthritis or the brevity of the duration between onset of arthritis and the uveitis, and (2) the severity of uveitis at initial presentation to the ophthalmologist.[5]

Rheumatologists try to take the broadest view of children who present with arthritis and/or uveitis. As pointed out by Schaller et al.,[3] the minority of juvenile arthritis patients with acute onset of uveitis are ANA-negative and turn out to have HLA-B27-positive ankylosing spondylitis or other spondyloarthropathies. But other rheumatologic diseases have been associated more rarely with uveitis, including vasculitis (Kawasaki's and Behcet's diseases) and granulomatous peri-arthritis (sarcoidosis). New attention is being paid to certain congenital connective tissue diseases associated with uveitis, namely those associated with mutations in CIAS1 (chronic neurologic, cutaneous and articular syndrome, or CINCA) and CARD15/NOD2 (Blau syndrome). Infection (Lyme disease, toxoplasmosis, Toxicara canis, tuberculosis) is always an important consideration in this population.

Pediatric rheumatologists see many children who present early in life, usually after 18 months of age, with knee arthritis. After ruling out Lyme disease, the toddlers who have persistent arthritis are universally referred for uveitis screening. Roughly 10% with uveitis turn out to have one of the spondyloarthropathies, which can be indistinguishable at presentation from the larger pauci-articular juvenile rheumatoid arthritis/JIA group. My experience has been that children with pauci-JRA more typically present with asymptomatic swelling in one or both knees, while kids with psoriatic arthritis have more painful involvement of the large joints of the lower extremities. The other spondyloarthropathies, particularly ankylosing spondylitis (AS) and reactive arthritis, more typically present after age 9.

Broadly speaking, uveitis tends to afflict roughly a third of pediatric AS and reactive arthritis patients, but fewer than 10% of inflammatory bowel disease or psoriatic patients. Presence of the HLA-B27 gene, which is expressed in about 8% of normal Caucasian children, is substantially overrepresented among these spondyloarthropathy patients who go on to develop uveitis.

The disease classification terminology regarding the major forms of childhood arthritis has been in a state of flux for several years, as rheumatologists in Europe and the U.S. have tried to reach consensus. This classification dilemma has ramifications for studies on uveitis in juvenile arthritis patients. In 1995, the International League Against Rheumatism (ILAR) proposed revised criteria for childhood arthritis, updated in 1997, that led to replacement of the Juvenile Rheumatoid Arthritis (JRA) designation used in the U.S. and the Juvenile Chronic Arthritis (JCA) term used in Europe. Criteria for these two entities were combined and validated with a new name, Juvenile Idiopathic Arthritis (JIA)—meaning childhood arthritis of unknown cause.

Some childhood arthritis subtypes are not uncommonly accompanied by uveitis. The oligoarthritis subtype is generally associated with a good prognosis for the joints, and is managed with non-steroidal anti-inflammatory agents (ie. ibuprofen, naproxen), intra-articular steroid injections, and occasionally disease modifying agents like methotrexate. The psoriatic arthritis subtype has a more challenging prognosis, with more frequent chronicity of the joint disease, and a greater reliance on methotrexate and anti-TNF biologic drugs like infliximab and adalimumab. The enthesitis-associated arthritis subtype, which overlaps with ankylosing spondylitis, is often treated with sulfasalazine and is increasingly met with early introduction of the anti-TNF drugs.

The one major therapeutic consideration in our arthritis patients with uveitis is the avoidance of the most popular anti-TNF drug, etanercept, which appears not to be effective in the treatment of uveitis.[6,7] The comparable efficacy of other drugs in the class (infliximab and adalimumab) against arthritis, and their substantial advantages in treating uveitis, make them a preferable choice for patients with both eye and joint manifestations. Other new therapies for arthritis are under consideration as potential treatments for refractory JIA-associated uveitis, including a longer-acting anti-TNF drug (certulizumab), a T-cell co-stimulation modulator (abatacept), a B-cell depletion drug (rituximab), and an IL6 antagonist (tocilizumab). The use of anti-IL1 therapy (anakinra) is under study in the congenital uveitis of CINCA and Blau syndrome.

With regard to uveitis screening in arthritis patients, the American Academy of Pediatrics has offered a set of suggested guidelines.[8] Children with arthritis onset before age 7 who are ANA-positive should be screened every 3 months. Less frequent screening (perhaps every six months) is appropriate if the ANA is negative, or the child had onset after age 7. Uveitis is very uncommon in children with the systemic form of JIA, and screening is not necessary on more than an annual basis.

There remains considerable controversy with regard to how many years this screening should continue, particularly in children who have repeatedly normal exams and subsequently resolve their arthritis. Caution and prudence are competing virtues in determining how best to prevent the devastating complication that loss of vision represents in some children with arthritis.

References:

1. Ohm J. Bandförmige Hornhauttrübung bei einem neunjährigen Mädchen und ihre Behandlung mit subkonjunktivalen Jodkaliumeinspritzungen. *Klin Monatsbl Augenheilhd* 1910;48:243-6.
2. Sury B. Rheumatoid arthritis in children. A clinical study.(thesis). Copenhagan: Munksgaard, 1952.
3. Schaller JG, Johnson GD, Holborow EJ, Ansell BM, Smiley WK. The association of antinuclear antibodies with chronic iridocyclitis of juvenile rheumatoid arthritis (Still's disease). *Arthritis Rheum.* 1974;17:409-416.
4. Rosenberg AM. Uveitis Associated with Juvenile Idiopathic Arthritis: Envisioning the Future. *J Rheum* 2002;29 (11):2253-5
5. Dana MR, Merayo-Lloves J, Schaumberg DA, Foster CS. Visual outcomes prognosticators in juvenile rheumatoid arthritis-associated uveitis. *Ophthalmol* 1997;104:236-44.
6. Foster CD, Tufail F, Waheed NK, Miserocchi E, Baltatzis S, Vredeveld CM. Efficacy of etanercept in preventing relapse of uveitis controlled by methotrexate. *Arch Ophthalmol* 2003;121(4):437-40
7. Smith JA, Thompson DJ, Whitcup SM, Suhler E, Clarke G, Smith S, Robinson M, Kim J, Barron KS. A randomized, placebo-controlled, double-masked clinical trial of etanercept for the treatment of uveitis associated with juvenile idiopathic arthritis. *Arthritis Rheum.* 2005;53:18-23.
8. Petty RE, Smith JR, Rosenbaum JT. Arthritis and uveitis in children: A pediatric rheumatology perspective. *Am J Opthalmol.* 2003;135:879-884.

Chapter 8
The Ophthalmologist Perspective

C. Stephen Foster, M.D., F.A.C.S., F.A.C.R.

Pediatric uveitis represents a serious issue in the ophthalmology community, and much of this topic has already been discussed in the previous sections of this monograph. Many of the challenges faced by uveitis specialists in managing childhood uveitis include delay in diagnosis, burden of the disease over a lifetime, difficulty with examinations, limited treatment options in children, and the risk of amblyopia. It is an enormous problem that is underappreciated worldwide, representing 10% of all uveitis cases. And yet it is responsible for 33% of legal blindness attributable to uveitis because these cases are not being followed long enough – and I emphasize the key phrase "followed long enough". Various publications on morbidities relating to pediatric ocular inflammatory disease often state that outcomes are not particularly bad, but when one looks at the follow up times for these studies, they only go as far as one, five, or ten years. The thirty year outcomes are exceedingly more discouraging.

Juvenile idiopathic arthritis (JIA; also juvenile rheumatoid arthritis or juvenile chronic arthritis) is the most common form of chronic arthritis in children and the most common systemic association with uveitis. About a third of such patients are treated in a tertiary uveitis setting. Typically the uveitis is a bilateral nongranulomatous anterior uveitis with onset before age 4 and is usually preceded by arthritis; however 10% of cases precede systemic symptoms and the uveitis does not correspond to the level of systemic disease at all.

How does JIA uveitis blind? There are multiple associated permanent complications which occur in patients with JIA-associated uveitis, and there are data from various clinics in the United States and Europe regarding these tragedies. Thorne and associates[1] reported the prevalence of complications as of 2007: cataract (19-81%), band keratopathy (7-75%), posterior synechiae (8-75%) (*Figures 1 and 2*), glaucoma (8-38%), macular edema (30%), and hypotony (19%).

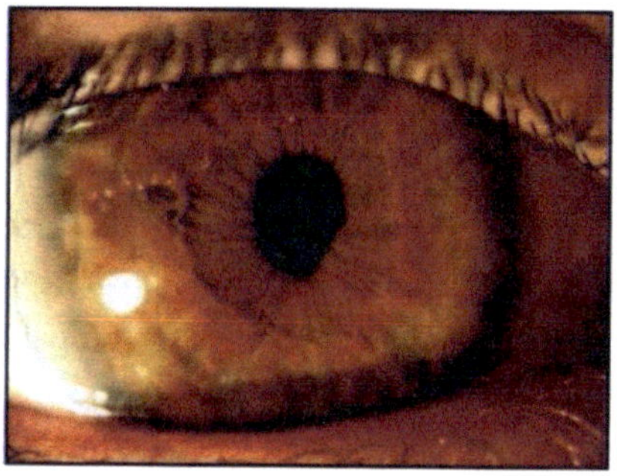

Figure 1

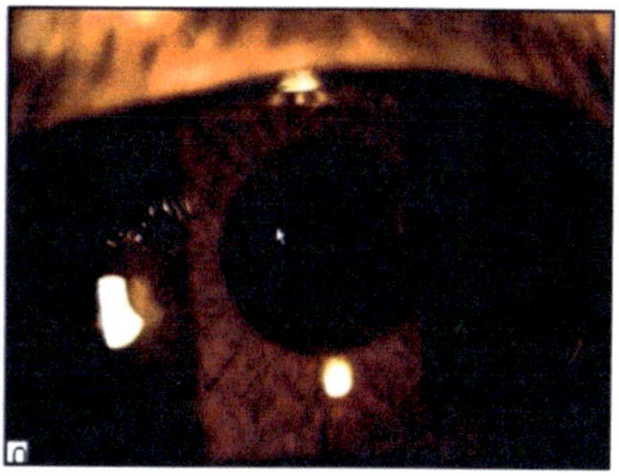

Figure 2

The complication rates are depressing when looked at year after year, with the incidence of any ocular complication near 0.33 per eye-year. The damage is cumulative, and while joint and skin inflammation may resolve, the eye generally ends with permanent damage and vision loss. The Rosenberg group demonstrated in 2004 in Miami[2] that higher numbers of significant vision-threatening complications increase with duration of disease and increasing follow up time, shown to occur in up to 86.3% of cases three years after presentation to an ophthalmologist. Woreta and colleagues reviewed 75 patients in Baltimore in 2007[3], and showed that 67% already had complications by the time the consultant was reached, featuring poor vision due to development of problems such as cataract, band keratopathy, and glaucoma. Almost 25% of the children were already legally blind at the time of first visit with the uveitis consultant.

I want to share with you now a case of a 10 year old girl with a 4 year history of bilateral uveitis that had been treated serially with topical steroids and regional steroid injections. She developed glaucoma and retinal problems requiring laser in both eyes. She had glaucoma surgery in the left eye and subsequent cataract formation. She was on topical corticosteroid, topical cyclosporine (an ill-conceived initiative to treat uveitis), and dilating and glaucoma medications. All along, her uveitis was poorly controlled, with numerous flares, treated only with corticosteroids repeatedly, when she finally presented to us at the Massachusetts Eye Research and Surgery Institution in Cambridge. She had hand motion vision in the left eye, and high pressure with active uveitis in the right eye – the better eye. The view to the retina was poor on the left as the tube from her valve had eroded through her cornea (Figure 3). Her mother had begged the child's uveitis "expert" for steroid-sparing, remission-inducing therapy. Her uveitis expert (not trained by fellowship) scorned this in fear of drug-related complications, calling this idea "reckless". Her pediatric ophthalmologist was a good advocate, urging the glaucoma specialist to fix her tube prior to possible infection. The glaucoma specialist, however, very wary of a risky procedure in an eye with "no visual potential", declined.

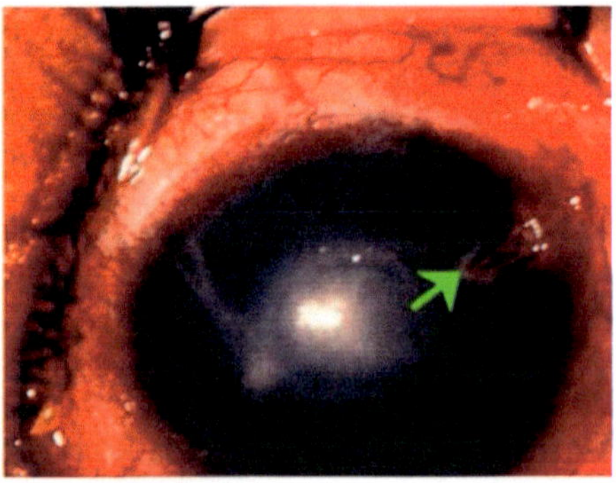

Figure 3 – Full thickness erosion of glaucoma shunt tube through peripheral cornea.

What would you do in this situation if this were your child? Would you leave it as is? Would you operate? And would you alter her medications or just continue the corticosteroid therapy? Imagine, for a moment, that this is your child. What would you wish for her care?

We operated, preserved and repositioned the valve, repaired her corneal defect, removed her cataract without artificial lens implant, and performed a complete vitrectomy. We left her aphakic, not wanting to put an intraocular lens inside an eye that had been through so much. Immediately after surgery, the patient was able to count fingers, her pressure was 5mm Hg, the eye was comfortable, and she finally began methotrexate therapy. Her family stayed until support for this mode of therapy at home was set up. Afterward, a vitrectomy was also performed in the right eye for increased inflammation. Eventually, the patient was 20/25 right eye and 20/60 left eye on a modest dose of methotrexate and her glaucoma was under control.

This story illustrates the burden of uveitis experts around the world – delayed referral and the discouragement of other doctors in giving referral even when asked. It is sad that today, in 2010, many children are not getting correct care and are irrevocably losing vision.

There are risk factors identified by various groups which predict a poor prognosis for children with uveitis – some that are very clear, and some still left for debate. Obvious risk factors include increased severity of uveitis at presentation, eye inflammation prior to joint inflammation, as well as prolonged interval of disease prior to seeing a uveitis specialist. [1,4-7] Gender has not yet been definitely shown to have an impact. Thorne and associates[1] showed that implementing steroid-sparing immunomodulatory therapy (IMT) early reduces the risk of ocular complications and blindness. Sabri and colleagues in Toronto in 2008[8] showed that many patients with a high prevalence of complications in eyes with uveitis were already legally blind by the time they were seen by a specialist. At my practice in Cambridge in 2006, 18% of children were already legally blind at presentation[9]. Thorne and associates in Baltimore[1] showed 25% were blind at first consultation, while the Rosenberg group in Miami[2] showed similar numbers. Smith and associates[10] showed slightly more than 9% of their patients presented with legal blindness. Different centers have different data, representing different treatment styles, referral patterns, and levels of aggressive treatment. Overall through the studies, about 10% of children with uveitis are legally blind at presentation to a uveitis specialist, and at one year, 5 years, and 10 years of delayed referral, the numbers are increasingly depressing.

So how does one attempt to modify the poor prognosis in children with JIA-associated uveitis? Early diagnosis is obvious and critical. The real challenge is finding the problem when ocular inflammation occurs before joint involvement. The only thing I can conceive to at least attempt to remedy this, perhaps, is legally mandated vision screening in preschools and in schools. There is no other way to detect the children with uveitis, no other trigger for evaluation besides reassessment of the current screening guidelines. For rheumatologists and pediatricians seeing children with JIA, the standard of care should be early referral to an ophthalmologist for uveitis screening. I have found rheumatologists are usually good at this, but I am not so sure about pediatricians, as there are still many late referrals. When the ophthalmologist sees uveitis, treating with corticosteroid therapy at first is correct, while following the problem closely to see how it responds to treatment. Monitoring must be done correctly until inflammation resolves. If and when inflammation recurs, the child is put back on corticosteroid therapy, which is correct – but how long is this cycle continued before referring? So often, referral is delayed for far too long, a major issue. I suggest referral to a uveitis specialist at the first recurrence.

The identification of high risk children has value. If a collection of features are identified that experts agree typify high-risk for stubborn or severe cases, these children should be treated more aggressively earlier with immunomodulatory therapy, before any complications develop. Once complications occur, the opportunity is lost to make a difference in the future for these children. I advise that the pediatrician and/or rheumatologist do whatever it takes to get the child to a real expert, a fellowship trained ocular immunologist. The referring doctor should be pro-active and co-manage the case with that expert, especially if the child lives far from the consultant.

The goal must be to eliminate all inflammation and limit exposure to corticosteroids. This involves a ladder approach with multiple steps. I treat aggressively with topical corticosteroids and with dilation. A periocular injection may help if the uveitis is more posterior, which may require sedation. If corticosteroids are required for more than 3 months, another path must be taken. Oral daily non-steroidal anti-inflammatory drugs (NSAIDs), such as naproxen or tolmetin, may prevent uveitis recurrence with steroid tapering and discontinuation[11]. But many patients with JIA-associated uveitis will need IMT, and they will need this for a minimum of two years off all steroids with no re-currences in order to be considered for tapering of the IMT, i.e., one should not be tempted to reduce IMT prior to two years in remission. Methotrexate is not the only available drug; there are many safe and effective immunomodulatory therapies that have been clinically shown to effectively treat uveitis, and several still needing future trials that have been widely agreed upon as effective. If methotrexate is not in-ducing corticosteroid-free remission, one should move along. Seventy-five percent of JIA-associated uveitis patients will respond to metho-trexate and be in remission, but 25% will not; these patients must move to other forms of IMT. Other similar anti-metabolite drugs like azathioprine and mycophenolate mofetil may work, as may other drugs which help to modify the cascade of signals involved in regulating in-flammatory cells, like cyclosporine. Alkylating drugs, such as cyclo-phosphamide and chlorambucil, are the most potent agents used and are extremely effective, but care must be taken as they have the most dangerous potential side effects, and should be monitored carefully while used in a limited number of children. Biologic response modifi-ers (BRMs), such as infliximab and adalimumab, may also be of bene-fit. This last category represents many of the emerging ideas for the treatment of uveitis worldwide. BRMs are not better drugs; they are just different – a different weapon in the fight against inflammation.

There is an urgent need for a set of therapeutic guidelines for treating pediatric uveitis, as well as uveitis in general.

Lastly, the coordination among caregivers for the diagnosis and management of pediatric uveitis is critical, especially when it comes to regular monitoring and examinations for children receiving IMT. A team approach between the ophthalmologist, rheumatologist, primary care physician and all other involved providers should be employed to help every affected child achieve the highest potential vision throughout their lifetime.

Summary of action items

- Establishment of standardized vision screening for children in schools
- Identification of children at risk for developing arthritis (i.e. JIA) and early referral to ocular immunologist
- Education to providers about immediate referral for patients with chronic or recurrent uveitis
- Awareness of need for lifetime follow-up for children with pediatric uveitis
- Education on avoidance of chronic use of topical or systemic corticosteroid therapy
- Development of therapeutic guidelines for treatment of stubborn cases of uveitis with immunomodulatory therapy to achieve durable steroid-free remission for no less than two years
- Coordination between providers during long-term management of children with uveitis

References

1. Thorne JE et al. Juvenile idiopathic arthritis-associated uveitis: incidence of ocular complications. *Am J Ophthalmol.* 2007; 143(5): 840-6.
2. Rosenberg KD, Feuer WJ, Davis JL. Ocular complications of pediatric uveitis. *Ophthalmol.* 2004;111(12): 2299-306.
3. Woreta F, et al. Risk factors for ocular complications and poor visual acuity at presentation among patients with uveitis associated with juvenile idiopathic arthritis (JIA). *Am J Ophthalmol.* 2007;143(4): 647-55.
4. Chia A, et al. Factors related to severe uveitis at diagnosis in children with juvenile idiopathic arthritis in a screening program. *Am J Ophthalmol.* 2003; 135(6): 757-62.
5. Dana MR, Merayo-Lloves J, Schaumberg DA, Foster CS. Visual outcomes prognosticators in juvenile rheumatoid arthritis-associated uveitis. *Ophthalmol* 1997; 104(2): 236-244.
6. Edelsten C, et al. Visual loss associated with pediatric uveitis in english primary and referral centers. *Am J Ophthalmol.* 2003;135(5), 676-80.
7. Edelsten C, et al. An evaluation of baseline risk factors predicting severity in juvenile idiopathic arthritis associated uveitis and other chronic anterior uveitis in early childhood. *Br J Ophthalmol.* 2002; 86: 51-6.
8. Sabri K, et al. Course, complications, and outcome of juvenile arthritis–related uveitis. *J AAPOS.* 2008 December; 12(6): 539-45.
9. Kump LI, Castaneda RA, Androudi SN, Reed GF, Foster CS. Visual outcomes in children with juvenile idiopathic-associated uveitis. *Ophthalmol.* 2006; 113(10): 1874-7.
10. Smith JA, Mackensen F, Sen HN, et al. Epidemiology and course of disease in childhood uveitis. *Ophthalmol.* 2009; 116(8): 1544-51.
11. Lee DH, Daud U, Wipfl J, Pepmueller PH, Davitt BV, Moore TL. The decreasing prevalence of uveitis associated with juvenile rheumatoid arthritis: do NSAIDs play a role? *J Clin Rheumatol.* 2003; 9(3): 151-5.

Chapter 9
Childhood Arthritis and Rheumatology Research Alliance: CARRA

C. Egla Rabinovich MD, MPH

CARRA stands for Childhood Arthritis and Rheumatology Research Alliance. CARRA is a research network of Pediatric Rheumatologists and Health Care Professionals dedicated to improving the treatment and outcomes of children with rheumatic diseases through investigator initiated clinical research. In order to study pediatric rheumatic disease, we need multicenter collaboration, as in rare diseases no one site has enough subjects to achieve meaningful significance. There are many unanswered questions in pediatric rheumatology that are important to doctors as well as families of children with rheumatic disease that will not be addressed by traditional funding mechanisms. For example, what are the long term outcomes of children with arthritis, what are the best treatments for childhood arthritis or uveitis?

Why do we need a research network for investigator initiated studies? We need to use the research network to improve the standard of care and promote a "culture" of research at Pediatric Rheumatology sites. The pediatric oncologists (cancer doctors) have shown us that children treated in protocols have better outcomes. They have been able to decrease mortality (deaths) from childhood cancers from about 80% in the 1950's to 20% by the use of cooperative research studies.

The mission of CARRA is: To prevent, treat and cure rheumatic diseases in children and adolescents through fostering, facilitating and conducting high quality research. The vision is that for all children with rheumatic diseases, CARRA will: perform clinical trials to define optimal care; conduct research that will translate to prevention, better treatment, and cure; investigate methods to improve quality of life in children; and promote a culture where all children will participate in research protocols. To achieve our mission and vision, CARRA will provide every child with a rheumatic disease in the United States (US) and Canada with the opportunity to participate in a study protocol by 2012.

CARRA has an organizational structure that includes an elected steering committee, 304 members, disease specific subgroups, and external advisory committee, a parent organization (Friends of CARRA), a finance committee and a nominations committee. Most pediatric rheumatology centers in the United States and Canada belong to this organization. There is a CARRA site map available on the CARRA website (CARRAgroup.org). CARRA is unique in that it is extremely collaborative. There is education, training and mentoring of members and sites (which is considered essential for network viability) through the annual meeting for members. At this meeting committees meet to prioritize, develop and foster studies. The goal is that each disease specific committee develops a portfolio of investigations, both observational and therapeutic. At this meeting there is an emphasis on dissemination of information, education regarding conduct of research, mentoring and new advances in science and protocol development. There are many opportunities to network, which is extremely important for the smaller sites where there may be only one pediatric rheumatologist. CARRA has a formalized written plan for sharing of data, specimens, study related tools and procedures.

CARRA was formed in 2002, and in the last eight years has made great strides. First a scientific agenda was developed for which there is an ongoing process for updating. We designed a protocol evaluation process as well as a site evaluation and performance process. We have held annual meetings since 2005. We were able to acquire infrastructure funding for the administrative core from the Arthritis Foundation (AF) for 2002-2010. We have 19 active studies funded by NIH-NIAMS

(National Institute of Health-National Institute of Arthritis and Musculoskeletal and Skin Diseases), AF, Friends of CARRA, Muscular Dystrophy Association, Mayo Foundation, Wegener's Granulomatosis Foundation, Shriner's Foundation, Pfizer, FDA and Alliance for Lupus Research. We had successful funding of Challenge Grant and Grand Opportunity grants from the NIH in 2009. Recent trials include:

- APPLE: Atherosclerosis Prevention in Pediatric Lupus Erythematosus
- TREAT: Trial of Early Aggressive Therapy in poly JIA
- RAPPORT: Randomized Placebo Phase study of Rilonacept in the Treatment of Systemic JIA
- RIM: Rituxan in Myositis
- Multicenter Prospective Registry of Infliximab Use for Childhood Uveitis:1st CARRA funded protocol
- Rilonacept in refractory Familial Mediterranean Fever

Future plans for enhancement of CARRA include development of a centralized Institutional Review Board (IRB) to decrease start-up time for trials, a common contract for sites, a centralized Data Center, increased site support for the research coordinator and site principal investigator, and inclusion of adult rheumatology groups. The latter is important since it has been recognized that up to half of all children with rheumatic diseases are cared for by adult rheumatologists.

In summary, CARRA has provided pediatric rheumatologists with a format for collaborative investigator initiated studies. Pediatric uveitis could benefit from a similar effort, or join with CARRA to study best treatments for pediatric uveitis as well as determination of long term outcomes. Pediatric uveitis, which is often treated by a team of ophthalmologists and rheumatologists, is a relatively rare disease where there remain many unanswered questions and thus would be an ideal area for partnering with CARRA.

Chapter 10

Pediatric Uveitis: Progress (or Lack Thereof) over the Past 20 Years

H. Nida Sen, MD, MHSc

Pediatric uveitis accounts for about 2.2 to 13.8% of patient visits in uveitis clinics[1]. It is well known that uveitis in children can have severe consequences, with great potential for vision loss. Delay in diagnosis, young age of onset, difficulty with examination and risks of adverse events from treatments all add to this potential. Thus, early use of systemic therapy is usually indicated. Several large cohorts have pointed to the high prevalence of complications among children with uveitis at the time of first diagnosis, along with the increasing prevalence in the few years after, inevitably resulting in high rates of vision loss[1-4].

In multiple studies over the last decade, the prevalence of complications in pediatric uveitis has ranged from 20% to 76%. The differences in methodology of these studies, however, make it difficult to ascertain whether the discrepancy in the rates of complications truly reflects a change in outcomes with time. In the past decade, the advent of newer forms of corticosteroid-sparing agents has changed the treatment approach in pediatric uveitis. It is still unclear whether this has resulted in fewer complications and improved visual outcomes.

One such study aimed to analyze the changes in treatment trends over 25 years and to compare visual outcomes, ocular surgeries performed, and complications of pediatric uveitis patients; specifically those treated in the 1980s or before, and those treated in the 1990s or after. The clinical records of all outpatients with pediatric uveitis (ages 0-18) with at least one visit before August 2005 with at least one follow-up appointment at three major tertiary care centers between 1955 and 1999 were investigated by Smith and associates[1]. The entire cohort could be divided into two groups based on the date of the first visit, the 1980s group and the 1990s group.

There were 64 patients in the 1980s cohort and 463 in the 1990s cohort. Systemic steroids were used in 30.6% of patients in the 1980s cohort and 43.6% in the 1990s cohort. NSAIDs were utilized in 4.8% and 14.2% of patients in each cohort. Similarly, the use of conventional immunosuppressives was 4.8% in the 1980s whereas it increased to 29.9% in the 1990s. Use of biologic response modifiers was 0% in the 1980s compared to 6.7% in the 1990s consistent with their availability.

In the 1980s cohort 35% of patients had vision ≥20/40 compared with 44% in the 1990s. The proportion of visual acuity outcomes that were legally blind cases was insignificantly less in the 1990s cohort (7% versus 12%, $p \leq -0.22$). The percentage of patients with any ocular complication and any ocular surgery was slightly higher in the 1990s cohort although the difference was not significant.

The results from this study demonstrate a clear trend in the wider use of systemic immunosuppressives in the last two decades. This trend has not, however, resulted in a decrease in complication rates or a significant improvement in visual outcomes. Whether this reflects a true increase in complications or stems from an ascertainment bias with the increased awareness and technology to detect complications is unclear. Long term prospective studies are clearly needed to evaluate whether more aggressive treatment strategies do indeed result in better outcomes.

References:

1. Smith JA, Mackensen F, Sen HN, Leigh JF, Watkins AS, Pyatetsky D, Tessler HH, Nussenblatt RB, Rosenbaum JT, Reed GF, Vitale S, Smith JR, Goldstein DA.Epidemiology and course of disease in childhood uveitis. *Ophthalmol.* 2009; 116(8):1544-51
2. Rosenberg KD, Feuer WJ, Davis JL. Ocular complications of pediatric uveitis. *Ophthalmol.* 2004; 111(12):2299-306.
3. Kump LI, Cervantes-Castañeda RA, Androudi SN, Foster CS. Analysis of pediatric uveitis cases at a tertiary referral center. *Ophthalmol.* 2005; 112(7):1287-92.
4. Thorne JE, Woreta F, Kedhar SR, Dunn JP, Jabs DA. Juvenile idiopathic arthritis-associated uveitis: incidence of ocular complications and visual acuity loss. *Am J Ophthalmol.* 2007;143(5):840-846.
5. Petty RE, Smith JR, Rosenbaum JT. Arthritis and uveitis in children. A pediatric rheumatology perspective. *Am J Ophthalmol.* 2003;135(6):879-84. Review.

Chapter 11
Consensus and a call to action

C. Stephen Foster, M.D., F.A.C.S., F.A.C.R.

This monograph was part of an effort to assess consensus among experts and to create an action item list in the approach to pediatric uveitis. The consensus would be on screening strategies, preferred practice patterns, future efforts, and a call to action to see if we can make a difference in the prevalence of blindness and visual disability secondary to pediatric uveitis over the next decade. Of course this has much to do with efforts such as those of CARRA and other collaborative studies. Finally, there would be plans to repeat this exercise 10 years from now to update the field on the most recent accomplishments in the management and treatment of pediatric uveitis – a reassessment of progress in 2020.

I felt that the easiest way to assess consensus was through use of a questionnaire, given to the physician speakers who participated in the conference on which this monograph was based, with answers tallied and used to evaluate the range of opinions on different issues. Questions were true or false type and were initially aimed at gauging the general conception of current preferred practice patterns, followed by an assessment of perceived risk factors for the chronicity or recurrence of juvenile idiopathic arthritis- (JIA) associated uveitis (Figure 1).

Though many such risk factors are well known and have been studied extensively, the risk factors for those cases likely to lead to severe or prolonged disease in patients with JIA-associated uveitis are not completely agreed upon. For example, it is clear in the evidenced-based literature that the pauciarticular or oligoarticular onset form of JIA carries a higher risk of uveitis development[1,2]. Does earlier age of onset or presence of uveitis at the time of initial presentation portend an increased risk of severity? One of the earliest published suspected risk factors was that of the presence of posterior synechiae at initial evaluation[3]. Though seemingly simple, this feature has stood the test of time among many uveitis specialists, i.e., patients with posterior synechiae at initial evaluation consistently are observed to have stubborn uveitis with a prolonged course. Some risk factors, such as gender and ANA positivity, have been debated. The presence of HLA-B27 haplotype is becoming more prominent in discussions surrounding prognosis of children with JIA-associated uveitis as an additional risk factor on top of those previously mentioned. A personal or even a family history of psoriasis and the presence of the HLA-DR5 allele have also been the subject of investigations and suspicion of conferring additional risk burden.

After tabulation of the answers to the questionnaire, the experts unanimously agreed that childhood uveitis is a vision-robbing problem of underappreciated importance, and that JIA-associated uveitis was the most prevalent form. They also agreed that about 75% of children with JIA-associated uveitis require long-term therapy for chronic or recurrent disease, and that continuous use of steroid therapy is not the accepted standard of care by specialists who manage patients with uveitis. Oligoarticular onset arthritis was also believed by all the experts to be a proven risk factor for chronic or recurrent uveitis.

Other possible risk factors were not unanimously agreed upon. All but one specialist agreed that uveitis onset at or prior to age 2 is a risk factor for severe or prolonged uveitis, as is the presence of posterior synechiae. Five of seven experts thought that uveitis onset prior to arthritis has been adequately shown to be a predictor of chronic or severe disease. A split exists in the literature between those who believe that either male or female gender presents a greater risk for a stubborn or difficult case, with reports showing clear evidence supporting both possibilities. ANA-positivity, while not completely agreed upon, was generally acknowledged as being a risk factor, reflecting the opinion of most experts. Five of seven experts agreed that the HLA-B27 allele as well as a personal or family history of psoriasis have not been shown in the literature to be a risk factor for having uveitis or for having it become chronic or recurrent, though these are things that are worth paying additional attention to going forward; the same applies to the HLA-DR5 allele.

Can we see a way now to push forward toward decreasing the prevalence of blindness in children with uveitis? Clearly education is critical, and especially the education of physicians. The specialists who have contributed to this monograph have made this their mission in life – teaching in residency programs, publishing in medical journals, attending and lecturing at Continuing Medical Education (CME) courses; and yet still we face the problem that is the subject of this monograph. There may not be the kind of emphasis on the subject of uveitis that is needed in the various residency programs of specialties which deal with pediatric uveitis patients. As Dr. Samson showed in his section, there is clearly a deficiency in ophthalmology residencies; only half, of ophthalmology residency programs in the United States have a part of their academic program dedicated to uveitis. And there is a dearth of uveitis specialists; only 12 of 132 ophthalmology residency training programs have a fellowship-trained and dedicated uveitis specialist on faculty. This means that every year the majority of another class of residents is exposed only to corticosteroids as a method to treat patients with uveitis, with no mentor to introduce them to alternative strategies. Rheumatology and pediatric residency training programs likely also lack emphasis on this matter.

Increased educational efforts are certainly needed, with contributions from the American College of Rheumatology (ACR), the American Academy of Ophthalmology (AAO), and the American Academy of

Pediatrics (AAP), as well as additional CME courses. One day prior to the yearly AAO meeting is "subspecialty day", which used to include only the major subspecialties such as cornea and retina. Happily, AAO has now adopted the more orphan subspecialties such as neurophthalmology and uveitis. It is encouraging that there is a full day dedicated to uveitis, which of course includes a section emphasizing management of pediatric uveitis as well.

Increased research efforts are also necessary. Is CARRA not the most logical resource for collaborative research on JIA? It makes sense to join and participate with CARRA from a research and an educational standpoint in order to make progress in this area. Consensus papers are important for several reasons, especially with respect to insurance company pushback toward use of expensive and off-label medications used in treating chronic and recurrent forms of uveitis. Typically these consensus papers evolve out of expert roundtable meetings; organizing such an event would be incredibly helpful toward achieving more success in these efforts.

Increased support and advocacy efforts should be made toward fostering better support of parents who seek the help of specialists in moving away from chronic corticosteroid therapy. There are many stories of the blockade that parents face in the advocacy of their children. The best course of action may be to educate physicians in order to avoid this tragedy, as well as making a better effort to listen to parents and allow them to effectively advocate for their child, rather than to discourage additional consultation or to discourage therapy with steroid-sparing medications. Lastly, ophthalmologists, specifically the American Uveitis Society, should reach out more toward other organizations such as the American Arthritis Foundation, insurance companies, and the CARRA group to emphasize just how truly important this topic remains throughout the world today.

Figure 1 – Questionnaire

1. Childhood uveitis is a vision-robbing problem of underappreciated importance.
2. JIA-associated uveitis is the most prevalent form of non-infectious pediatric uveitis.
3. Approximately 75% of children with JIA-associated require chronic or recurrent therapy for their uveitis which is chronic or recurrent.
4. Open ended chronic or recurrent corticosteroid therapy is an accepted standard of care approach to the treatment of childhood uveitis.
5. Which of the following are risk factors for a child's JIA-associated uveitis being chronic or recurrent?
    a. Oligoarticular-onset arthritis
    b. Uveitis onset at or before age 2
    c. Uveitis onset prior to arthritis onset
    d. Posterior synechiae present at first slit lamp examination
    e. Male patient
    f. Female patient
    g. ANA positive
    h. HLA-B27 positive
    i. Personal or family history of psoriasis
    j. HLA-DR5 positive

Figure 2 – Summary of action items

- Education about the importance of Pediatric Uveitis
    - American College of Rheumatology
    - American Academy of Pediatrics
    - American Academy of Ophthalmology

- Education about the importance of Ocular Immunology faculty
    - American University Professors of Ophthalmology
    - American Board of Ophthalmology
- Collaborative research – CARRA
- Consensus "white paper" production and publication
- Uveitis specialty society outreach/networking
- AAO preferred practice pattern for uveitis to be developed

References

1. Cassidy JT, Sullivan DB, Petty RE. Clinical patterns of chronic iridocyclitis in children with juvenile rheumatoid arthritis. *Arthritis and Rheum.* 1977; 20: 224-8.
2. Kanski JJ. Juvenile arthritis and uveitis. *Surv Am J Ophthalmol.* 1990; 34(4): 253-67.
3. Wolf MD, Lichter PR, Ragsdale CG. Prognostic factors in the uveitis of juvenile rheumatoid arthritis. *Ophthalmol.* 1987 Oct; 94(10): 1242-8.
4. Viera KA, et al. Male gender and poor visual outcomes in uveitis associated with juvenile idiopathic arthritis. *Am J Ophthalmol.* 2010; 149 (6): 987-993.
5. Heiligenhaus A. et al. Prevalence and complications of uveitis in juvenile idiopathic arthritis in a population-based nation-wide study in Germany: suggested modification of the current screening guidelines. *Rheumatol.* 2007; 6: 1015-9.
6. Zak M, Fledelius H, and Pedersen FK. Ocular complications and visual outcome in juvenile chronic arthritis: a 25-year follow-up study. *Acta Ophthalmol Scand.* 2003; 81: 211-5.
7. Kump LI, Castaneda RA, Androudi SN, Reed GF, Foster CS. Visual outcomes in children with juvenile idiopathic-associated uveitis. *Ophthalmol.* 2006; 113(10): 1874-7.
8. Woreta F, et al. Risk factors for ocular complications and poor visual acuity at presentation among patients with uveitis associated with juvenile idiopathic arthritis (JIA). *Am J Ophthalmol.* 2007; 143(4): 647-55.
9. Saurenmann RK, et al. Risk factors for development of uveitis differ between girls and boys with juvenile idiopathic arthritis. *Arthritis Rheum.* 2010; 62 (6): 1824-8.
10. Özdal PC, Vianna RNG, Deschênes J. Visual outcome of juvenile rheumatoid arthritis-associated uveitis in adults. *Ocul Immunol Inflamm.* 2005; 13: 33-8.

11. Yu EN, et al. Outcomes of treatment with immunomodulatory therapy in patients with corticosteroid-resistant juvenile idiopathic arthritis-associated chronic iridocyclitis. *Ocul Immunol Inflamm.*2005; 13: 353-60.
12. Kempen JH, et al. Methods for identifying long-term adverse effects of treatment in patients with eye diseases: The systemic immunosuppressive therapy for eye diseases (SITE) cohort study. *Ophthalmic Epidemiol.* 2008; 15: 47-55.
13. Thorne JE et al. Juvenile idiopathic arthritis-associated uveitis: incidence of ocular complications. *Am J Ophthalmol.* 2007; 143(5): 840-6.
14. Dana MR, Merayo-Lloves J, Schaumberg DA, Foster CS. Visual outcomes prognosticators in juvenile rheumatoid arthritis-associated uveitis. *Ophthalmol* 1997; 104(2): 236-244.
15. Rosenberg KD, Feuer WJ, Davis JL. Ocular complications of pediatric uveitis. *Ophthalmol.* 2004; 111(12): 2299-306.
16. Sabri K, et al. Course, complications, and outcome of juvenile arthritis–related uveitis. *J AAPOS.* 2008; 12(6): 539-45.
17. Kotaniemi K, et al. Occurrence of uveitis in recently diagnosed juvenile chronic arthritis – A prospective study. Ophthalmol. 2001;108 (11): 2071-5.

The Ocular Immunology and Uveitis Foundation is a 501c(3), not-for-profit, tax-exempt organization. Our mission is to find cures for ocular inflammatory diseases, to correct the worldwide deficit of properly trained ocular immunologists, and to provide education and emotional support for those patients afflicted with ocular inflammatory disease.

We Believe…

- In this day and age, no patients should suffer with poor treatment for ocular inflammatory disease.

- A cure is possible for ocular inflammatory disease.

- We can correct the deficit of properly trained ocular immunologists.

- Patients should have ample support during this time of need.

www.uveitis.org

Made in the USA
Monee, IL
05 November 2026

67381610R00050